FREED
CHEMICAL

By
Devi S. Nambudripad,
M.D., D.C., L.Ac., Ph.D.

Author of
Say Good-Bye To Illness and
Say Goodbye to ... Series of Books

This book has already revolutionized
THE PRACTICE OF MEDICINE

The doctor of the future will give no medicine,
But will interest his patients
In the care of the human frame, in diet,
And in the cause and prevention of disease
Thomas A. Edison

Published by
DELTA PUBLISHING COMPANY
6714 Beach Blvd.
Buena Park, CA 90621
(888)-890-0670, (714) 523-8900 Fax: (714)-523-3068
Web site: www.naet.com

DEDICATION

This book is dedicated to
All Chemically Sensitive patients, and
Any one wishing to get well through NAET

First edition, 2006

Library of Congress Control No: **2006934419**

ISBN: **09759277-8-7**

Printed in U.S.A.

Table of Contents

Acknowledgement vii

Foreword.. xi

Preface.. xvi

Introduction.. xxix

Chapter 1

MSG Sensitivity.. 1

Causes of Chemical Sensitivities..4

The Brain and the Nervous System... 8

The Nervous System 9

The Brain and Allergies..11

The Communication Network 13

NAET® Intervention 15

The Basis of NAET® 18

What is NAET®?...19

How was NAET® Discovered?..20

Overview of NAET® 21

Attraction Between Energies...25

Repulsion Between Energies..25

Natural Body Defense...26

Home Evaluation Procedures...28

Organ-Meridian Association Time...................... 30

Names of the Meridians 30

Meridian Clock 31

Allergy Symptom Checklist.....................................33

Chapter 2

What is Chemical Sensitivity? 47

What is Multiple Chemical Sensitivity? 48

Categories of Allergies 56

Inhalants 59

Ingestants 70

Contactants 76

Injectants 79

Infectants 80

Physical agents 82

Genetic Causes..83

Molds and Fungi...84

Emotional Stressors...86

A Case Study.. 87

Chapter 3

Detecting Allergies...89

Food Chemicals 94

Nambudripad's Testing Techniques.............................101

Chapter 4

Symptoms of Meridians 107
Normal Energy Flow Through 12 Meridians.........................108
Lung Meridian..109
Large Intestine Meridian..113
Stomach Meridian..115
Spleen Meridian...119
Heart Meridian...121
Small Intestine Meridian..123
Urinary Bladder Meridian..125
Kidney Meridian..127
Pericardium Meridian...129
Triple Warmer Meridian...131
Gall Bladder Meridian..133
Liver Meridian...135
Governing Vessel Meridian...137
Conception Vessel Meridian...139

Chapter 5

NAET® Testing Procedures 141
Neuromuscular Sensitivity Testing 143
NST without Allergen...144

Balancing the Body...144
NST with Allergen 148
NST Weak with Allergen...148
O Ring Testing...149
Testing Through a Surrogate..150
Finger on Finger Testing...151
Extended Surrogate Testing..152
A Tip to Master Self-testing 153
Testing for Person to Person Allergy....................................156
Question Response Testing 157
NST-QRT Procedures 158
Asking Questions 158
Technique of Asking Questions...159

Chapter 6

NAET® Home Help 163
About Testing 172
NAET® Basic Allergens..173
NAET Classic Allergens 173
Other Chemicals..188
Treating by Priority 192
Self-testing Procedures...192
Isolation Technique..196
Acutherapy...198

Points to Reduce Chemical Sensitivity..............................200

Acute Care..201

Oriental Medicine CPR Points...202

Resuscitation Points 203

Commonly Seen Emotional Blockages 205

Chapter 7

A Collection of Cases 207

Glossary...239

Resources...263

Bibliography..267

Index..277

Acknowledgment

I am deeply grateful to my husband, Kris Nambudripad, for his encouragement and assistance in my schooling and later, in the formulation of this project. Without his cooperation in researching reference work, revision of manuscripts, word processing and proofreading, it is doubtful whether this book would have ever been completed.

My sincere thanks also go to the many clients who have entrusted their care to me, for without them I would have had no case studies, no feedback, and certainly no extensive source of personal research upon which to base this book.

I am also deeply thankful to Helen Tanner, Karen Watts, Margaret Brazil, Jennifer Bentley, Lettie Vipond, Toby Weiss, Terri weiss, Amy Clute, Rosemary Depau, Margaret Davies, Barbara Cesmat, Jeanne Soriano, Nancy Molinari, Michael Mag, Jean E, Joan E, Debbie H., Bill H., Ron M., Martha Evans, Patty Hobbs, to name a few among many of my devoted patients, for believing in me from the very beginning of the research until the present, and by supporting my theory and helping me to conduct the ongoing detective work.

I also have to express my thanks to my son, Roy Nambudripad, MD, who assisted me in many ways in the writing of this book.

Additionally, I wish to thank Robert Prince, M.D., Laurie Teitelbaum, MS, Chi Yu, Fong Tien and many of my associates, who wish to remain anonymous for proofreading and assisting me with this work, and Mr. Sri at Delta Publishing for his printing expertise. I am deeply grateful for my professional training and the knowledge and skills acquired in classes and seminars on chiropractic and kinesiology at the Los Angeles College of Chiropractic in Whittier which is now called the Southern University of Health Sciences, California; the California Acupuncture College in Los Angeles; SAMRA University of Oriental Medicine, Los Angeles; University of Health Sciences, School of Medicine, Antigua; and the clinical experience obtained at the clinics attached to these colleges.

My special thanks also go to Mala Moosad, N.D., R.N., L.Ac., Ph.D., Mohan Moosad, M.S., N.D., D.Ac, who supported and stood by me from the very beginning of my NAET discovery and ongoing research. They helped immensely by taking over my work load at the clinic so that I could complete the book. I also would like to acknowledge my thanks to my dear mother for nourishing me forever emotionally and nutritionally. My heartfelt thanks also go to Dr. Marilyn Chernoff, Barbara Cesmat, Sister Naina, and Margaret Wu, NAET® trained practitioners, who have dedicated their time to help desperate allergy sufferers by assisting me in many ways to promote my mission of making NAET® available to every needy person not only in this country, but in third world countries as well. I would also like to acknowledge my everlasting thanks to my office manager, Janna Gossen, who worked with me from the first day of my practice of two decades and to Sarah Cardinas, Patty Hobbs, and Kathy Franklin for their support.

I would like to remember the late Dr. Richard F. Farquhar at Farquhar Chiropractic Clinic in Bellflower, California. I was a student of chiropractic and acupuncture when I was doing preceptorship with him. When I told him about my NAET® discovery, he tried the treatment on himself and was amazed with the results. Then he encouraged me to practice NAET® with needles on all his patients. Because of his generosity, I had the opportunity to treat hundreds of patients soon after I discovered NAET®.

I do not have enough words to express my heartfelt thanks and appreciation to the California Acupuncture State Board for supporting NAET® from the beginning, permitting me to teach other licensed acupuncturists by instantly making me a CEU provider. Perhaps the California Acupuncture State Board will never know how much they have helped humanity by validating my new technique and allowing me to share the treatment method with other practitioners and, through them, to the countless number of patients like me, who now live normal lives. I am forever indebted to acupuncture and Oriental medicine. Without this knowledge, I myself, would still be living in pain. Thank you for allowing me to share my experience with the world!

I am so delighted to express my sincere thanks to the Los Angeles College of Chiropractic for teaching different branches of holistic medicine like kinesiology and Sacrooccipital techniques along with chiropractic in our school and providing the students with a sound knowledge in nutrition. Because of that I was able to combine the art of kinesiology, chiropractic and nutrition along with acupuncture/acupressure and develop NAET®. California Acupuncture College also taught me a few lessons in kinesiology along with the art and science of acupuncture.

I also extend my sincere appreciation and thanks to my medical school professors for willing to part with their knowledge and help us become great physicians. I would like to extend my sincere thanks to these great teachers especially to my medical school mentors and professors from Antigua and from California, and the staff of the respective hospitals where I did my clinical rotations. Without their guidance and teaching I doubt if I could have completed the medical school.

All my mentors from all professional schools I attended have helped me to grow immensely at all levels. They are also indirectly responsible for the improvement of my personal health as well as that of my family, patients, and the health of other NAET® practitioners and their countless patients.

Many of my professors, doctors of Western and Oriental medicine, allopathy, chiropractic, kinesiology, as well as nutritionists, were willing to give of themselves by teaching and committing personal time, through interviews, to help me complete this book. I will always be eternally grateful to them. They demonstrated the highest ideals of the medical profession.

Devi S. Nambudripad,
M.D., D.C., L.Ac., Ph.D.(Acu.)
Los Angeles, California
October 2006

FOREWORD
By
Ann McCombs, D.O.

It is with great pleasure that I have been asked to write the Foreword to Dr. Devi's most recent book in her allergy series: Freedom from Chemical Sensitivities. While all of her books have been timely written and welcome additions to the field of Complementary and Alternative Medicine, I find this topic to be especially so, as toxicity is a factor in the lives of people everywhere and, especially, in the more industrially developed areas of the world. We are all at risk for these allergies, in one way or another, and the seriousness of this fact is appreciated (in my opinion) by a relative few. Expressed in a slightly different way:

What if you knew that the major cause of chemical sensitivities is environmental toxins and that, if left untreated, a large percentage of them would progress to cancer?

What if you knew that the hidden source of these acute and chronic chemical sensitivities lay in your body's inability to excrete these toxins faster than you can take them in, thus creating a toxic overload of such magnitude that ~ because they are predominantly stored in the fat cells of our bodies ~ they may be an as-yet-undiscovered cause of obesity in the industrial world?

What if you knew that one of the major underlying causes for such childhood afflictions as ADD, ADHD and autism may actually stem from the child's exposure to his/her mother's toxins in utero (especially if first-born), even before being exposed to childhood vaccines preserved with thimerasol (a mercury-containing compound) that have become practically mandatory in the western world?

What if you knew that the reason you (or your child, spouse, neighbor, friend, etc) have a constant runny nose, frequent colds, headaches, body aches that just won't resolve, etc (and, especially, in the face of all the test results being "normal") really was due to the "sick" building you work in every day or the newly-constructed school your child attends this year?

What if you knew that the latex gloves that "everybody" knows are harmless, or the formaldehyde in the particle board, "do-it-yourself" furniture all over your house, or the root canal filling material you had placed in your tooth 20+ years ago could render you as incapacitated as the boy in the bubble in the flash of that one additional exposure that really became the "straw that broke the camel's back"?

Would any of these scenarios make a difference in the attention you paid while reading a book such as this? Probably not...unless you have been touched ~ first-hand ~ by experiences such as these, as I and many others like me, have been.

As a holistic family physician, I can vouch for the truth of the above scenarios, because I treat the people/families to whom these outcomes have happened...and I have had my own seemingly "out of the box" experiences touted by some of my colleagues (even in the holistic medicine world, I'm sad to say) as being "preposterous, by any stretch of the imagination." However, since meeting Dr. Devi nearly 12 years ago now, my life has not been the same...nor have my patients' lives, I'm grateful to say. Not only did she bring hope and health back into my own life (and still does!), she has influenced me as a physician, inspired me as a colleague and supported me as a friend when I was deep in my own dark night of the soul, uncertain where to look next for answers for either myself or my patients. She is a true pioneer in the deepest sense of the word, and I am proud to be her student, colleague and friend…and, one day (in the not too distant future of the dot.com world, I trust), it is my fervent prayer that Dr. Devi will take her true place in the world of healing (notice: I did not say medicine!) and be recognized for her amazing, efficacious, non-invasive and cost-effective method (NAET®) which makes it possible now to truly say goodbye to not only multiple chemical sensitivities, but to all illnesses and dis-eases.

Thank you, dear Devi, from all of us who have been so deeply touched and forever changed by your many gifts and talents, not to mention your sweet spirit and gentle nature, even in the face of blatant attack by those who do not yet have eyes to see and ears to hear the different drummer and music which lifts your feet and to which you march, unfailingly and cheerfully, day by day, secure in who you are and your mission in this world. You're beautiful…and I'm proud to be part of your parade. Keep on keeping on, for all of us need what you know, both personally and professionally.

Ann McCombs, D.O.
Kirkland, WA
October 2006

PREFACE

I have suffered from numerous health problems since childhood. Because of this prolonged and firsthand ex perience with ill health, I became focused on health-related problems, particularly those related to allergies; this, in turn, resulted in my natural inclination to pursue medicine as a profession. Consequently, I became a registered nurse, chiropractor, kinesiologist, acupuncturist and earned a doctorate in philosophy in Oriental medicine. Then, I realized that I lacked one more degree which was quite essential for me to continue to teach internationally and help others. So I decided to return to traditional medical school and earned an MD degree. I have been in school all my life, searching for answers to help myself and others with health-related disorders. I began specializing in the treatment of the allergic patient, using methods I learned through an intensive study of Oriental medicine combined with the more traditional Western methods learned in various schools of Western medicine.

During my studies and early practice as an allergist, while using eclectic methods of allergy treatments, I discovered a technique that eliminated most of my health problems.

Integrating the relevant techniques from the various health fields I studied, combined with my own discoveries, this new treatment has become the focus of my practice. There is no known successful method of treatment for chemical sensitivities or allergies using Western medicine except avoidance, which means deprivation and frustration. Each of the disciplines I studied provided bits of knowledge that I used in developing a new treatment to permanently eliminate most of my chemical sensitivities and allergies. This treatment is now known throughout the world as Nambudripad's Allergy Elimination Techniques, or NAET® for short.

As an infant living in India, my birthplace, I had severe infantile eczema which lasted until I was seven or eight years old. My eczema started at 11 months old after eating a whole tomato one night instead of dinner, as my mother recalled. After that, I was administered Western medicine, Ayurvedic herbal medicine and various cleansing diets without a break until I was eight years old. In spite of all these efforts, my eczema continued. I was born and brought up as a vegetarian. From childhood, my major diet was organically grown vegetables, fruits and grains grown in our fields (without using any artificial or chemical fertilizers). My family was into farming. When I turned one year old, all of my health problems began one after another, after the memorable 'Tomato' dinner: It started as generalized skin rashes, hives, eczema, dermatitis, sinus troubles, infections, angioneurotic edema (swelling in different body parts–frequently eyelids, face, sometimes even throat without any warning or known cause), and severe arthritis. My saga continued... frequent colds and fevers, flu-like symptoms, constant post nasal drip, thick mucus in the throat, pain and swelling in the joints, severe fatigue, and general body aches. By the time I was ten, I began having severe migraines, then later, severe PMS. I never had anything mild. My symptoms were always in extremes making living difficult. I spend my childhood visiting doctors and taking medicines, yet I still suffered constantly.

After discovering NAET®, treating myself and eliminating all my known allergies, sensitivities to man-made chemicals still remained a big problem for me. Chemicals are hidden in many unexpected places around us. The major sources of chemicals that we encounter in our everyday lives are from our foods and household environments. These sources include: food chemicals such as food colorings, food additives, food preservatives, taste enhancers (MSG), appearance and texture enhancers, vegetables and fruits grown using chemical fertilizers and sprayed with various highly toxic pesticides either while growing or packaging, herbs and vitamins; water chemicals from polluted water (gray water, black water, etc.); oral or injectable drugs, immunizations and vaccinations; environmental chemicals such as pesticides, insecticides, chemical fertilizers, heavy metals, smoke and fumes from wood burning, exhaust, toxic waste from various sources, weather related conditions encouraging toxic releases in the environments, radon, and radiation, petrochemicals such as housewares, household cleansing chemicals, detergents, soaps, fabric softeners, beauty supplies and products, chemically treated fabrics, synthetic fabrics, dry cleaning agents, plastics and vinyl products, paper products, work and school related chemicals, etc. This list could go on and on since new man-made chemicals are being created daily.

Whenever I had an allergic reaction to a product I would read all the ingredients in the product. Sure enough there would be one or two items on the list that are totally new and that I had not treated for prior to the reaction. I would desensitize to the product immediately, thinking of and picturing the untreated items in my mind. I did not know how to get those particular chemicals isolated in its individual form anywhere for purchase. After the NAET® desensitization to the particular item(s), I usually felt better and after 25 hours, that particular item(s) did not bother me anymore. That was a great relief. The saddest thing was this: when I came across another untreated item, I reacted the same way. I thought I was wasting so much time in treating different chemicals. I could have done lots of other things in my life instead of spending time in NAET® treatments, but I had no choice. If I wanted to live normally among others I had to desensitize for the chemicals as they crossed my path. I tried to avoid all chemicals as much as I could. Even with avoidance, there is no guarantee that chemically sensitive people will be able to stay away from every possible chemical exposure and still remain reaction free. Initially, when I discovered NAET®, I thought I reacted to everything I touched and everything I came across. People around me did not have that kind of sensitivity. By then I had forgotten my miserable childhood days when I would spend days at a time in bed unable to get up from the bed. I had to be carried to the toilet on certain days. My joint pains were so bad, I couldn't even limp to the porch to peek at other children (my cousins) playing in the courtyard happily. Often I wondered why God brought me to earth to suffer in this fashion without showing any mercy.

We had a family tradition of celebrating every family member's birthday in my house including my parents' and grand-mothers'. All my four uncles followed the same tradition too. All of our four families, who lived a mile or so away from each other, would get together to celebrate everyone's birthday either in my house or theirs. For generations this tradition was maintained by my family. I think there was a reason behind that tradition. While I was growing up the caste system was still very predominant in the part of India where I grew up and the children from our families were not allowed to play with the children from other social groups from the neighborhood. The women from our families were not allowed to travel alone even to visit temples or to do any shopping. They had to be chaperoned no matter where they went. Girls after menarche were forced to stop their schooling if they had to travel to schools and sit in the class among other students. Home-schooling was permitted with women teachers only. (I was the first girl from my family who was able to break the tradition, move out of my house to another city to continue my education after I grew up). By arranging these frequent birthday celebrations, the isolated women of our families would get to meet other family members; women especially cherished these get togethers. They got the opportunity to meet our cousins, aunts and grandmothers and participate in the traditional group dance that was performed by women soon after lunch. The women and grown up children looked forward to these dances. Often our men joined in the dances. The children looked forward to these birthdays because they could also play the whole day with their cousins. We never had the custom of exchanging gifts or bringing food. The host family prepared delicious meals for everyone and everyone spent the entire day at home and left in the evening until the next occasion to meet in another house. Often I became sicker during those parties and remained in bed or sat quietly on a chair near the grown-up women listening to their jokes or group songs. Women from my family did not gossip those days. Probably, they did not have any time left to gossip. After the main meal at noon, they performed the special group dance and when they got exhausted from the dance they ate more food. Even though I was often sick, enjoyed eating all the goodies offered to me by my aunts. They offered me more food and they forced me to eat more; they took special interest to prepare my favorite dishes in order to cheer me up since often I couldn't take part in the dances or games the other children played. Now I can guess the cause of my nagging arthritic pains or headaches during those much awaited family get togethers. I must have been allergic to all the delicious snacks and special favorite foods I ate causing me to be sick during the following days or weeks after the party until the allergens had the chance to leave my body. Then of course in a couple of weeks we had another get together, repeating the whole scenario again thus keeping me in pain at least one half of the year.

Some of my uncles and aunts also suffered from similar kind of arthritic pains throughout the year. They also were on year-round herbal massages, herbal concoctions and medications hoping to find some relief from their on-going pains. No one talked about allergies; perhaps no one knew the concept of allergy. No one could imagine someone to be allergic to the same food that they began consuming almost daily from infancy and the very food that nourished them and helped them to grow into adulthood. They all believed that they had contracted some incurable disorders and never once gave up eating the delicious meals at the gatherings.

After I discovered NAET®, my days were much better than the days of my childhood. I had many days without pain even though I knew I had a long list of foods to be desensitized. After I treated for a few items, initially I was very happy thinking of the possibility of seeing the light at the end of the tunnel. I was ecstatic thinking that I had really discovered something big that could bring an end to so many people's pains. The good feeling didn't last too long. I began to react to everything around me. When I continued to react to various things without relief for several weeks, when my fibromyalgia and joint pains returned, when I began to notice or identify numerous chemicals that I reacted to from the foods I ate and my environment, I became sad, depressed, very impatient, irritable and frustrated. At that point the dream of having a normal life left me completely. I was unable to think normally; the only thing I could do was just cry. My emotions were very fragile. I avoided communication with my friends. I made excuses and didn't attend their parties and get-togethers when I was invited. I didn't wish to tell them about my health problems. No one was able to help me with my problems, not even the number of medical specialists I had seen in the past. The last thing I wanted from anyone was sympathy. I was going into a depression.

I am blessed with a caring, loving husband, who is wise and understanding. He observed me and my behavior silently for a few days. Then one day he told me very calmly to reevaluate my present situation. He reminded me that I was more fortunate than all others in the world who suffered from pain and other illnesses. When I reacted to an item, I knew how to detect the culprit in seconds using NAET® testing procedures; once detected it took several minutes only to desensitize myself for that item, never to have to worry about that reaction again, whereas many millions of people suffer from various types of pains and live in misery all the time without knowing why they were hurting or how to find a solution. "Yes, you have numerous allergies," he consoled me, "You can't get impatient and frustrated like this. Let's face one allergen at a time and treat them all. Soon you will be free from their clutches."

I was too emotional to resist him. So I followed his suggestion. I had two months summer vacation from school. (I was still a student at that time). My husband also took a month's vacation from his work. We stayed home and continued to treat two to three items a day, everyday and I avoided everything I treated so carefully for the following 25 hours. In about three weeks we had treated so many items that at last I began to see a difference in my reactions. My extreme reactions to the surrounding chemicals reduced. Once again my hopes returned to see the light at the end of the tunnel. The veil of depression began leaving me slowly.

It took me about a year (at one to two treatments a day) before I felt moderately comfortable to live again. After four years of hard work and continuous treatments, I reached the end of the tunnel waking up **to the brightest light anyone has ever seen. Yes, I was free from most allergies by then.**

With the progress of science and technology, our modern lifestyles have changed dramatically. New products, which are potential allergens for many people, are being developed every day. Scientists are out there spending their precious hours scratching their brains, staying up through early morning hours; they are searching for ways to bring out entirely new products into the market by the following week so that their products will be better than their competitors'. With the appearance of the new chemical products the quality of life has improved; but for some chemically sensitive people these scientific achievements have just created more nightmares.

We cannot ignore the fact that we are in the twenty-first century where technology is ever more predominant than before. There is nothing wrong with the technology. In fact, modern technology has provided a new avenue of comforts to many. But the allergic patient must find ways to overcome adverse reactions to chemicals and other allergens produced by this technology in order to enjoy living.

Even though it requires a series of detailed treatments, NAET® offers the prospect of relief to those who suffer from constant allergic reactions by reprogramming the brain to perfect health. Just like rebooting a computer, we can reboot our nervous systems through NAET® and overcome the adverse reactions of our brains and our bodies.

Many illnesses these days arise from our interactions with the toxins around us—the toxins produced from chemical products, sprays and fumes, the very substances we use to clean our bodies and environments, to beautify ourselves, to ward off insects, and to keep our environments clean and beautiful. We do all this in the hope of keeping ourselves healthy and happy. When these toxins turn against us, when we suffer the after effects and ill effects of using them, we become confused and helpless. Most of us find salvation from all of this in a doctor's office. A smart doctor will refer to your reactions by familiar medical names instead of calling you crazy (even though that is likely what he is thinking but isn't cruel enough to tell you to your face). This doctor may even recommend a medication that has helped his other patients who have had similar reactions. If we are lucky, our symptoms will be reduced or eliminated and we will feel better and continue with our lives until the next attack.

NAET® is a simple technique that involves art and science from various medical disciplines. According to NAET® theory, allergies are the result of energy blockages in the body that are triggered by contact with various allergens. These triggers may especially be chemicals from in and/or around the body. NAET® desensitization treatments can release these energy blockages from the specific areas of the meridians. It then can reprogram the brain not to react to the densitized substances adversely with future contacts. NAET® not only eliminates the allergy but it also balances the body's energetics and helps the body make the decision not to react to that allergen in the future.

In most cases, the person who gets treated with NAET® feels better and better after each treatment. It may take a couple of years for a person to become desensitized to every item on their long list of allergens, but in most cases, the patient begins to feel better right after the first treatment.

NAET® treatments prepare the brain to respond normally to the treated allergen. This does not mean that after treating for a harmful chemical, our body does not recognize that the chemical is dangerous or harmful When the body encounters the treated chemical in the future, the body releases it without causing panic or turmoil in the body.

Without knowing what is an allergen and what is not an allergen, we continue to expose ourselves to harmful allergens many times every day. Continuous exposures and re-exposures to various allergens throughout one's daily living can aggravate the condition of the body further. In such people, the presence of an allergen can trigger immediate allergic reactions, usually attacking the weakest organ first. Eventually, the other organs will be affected as well.

Our evolution is the probable cause for the high prevelance of allergies these days. Our ancestors had different health problems such as bacterial infections and parasitic infestations. There were not so many chemicals or environmental hazards during those times. Their bodies were trained to overcome and live with the problems they had and their genes carried the messages of survival into the genes of their descendants (our genes). However, the genes of our ancestors were never exposed to the thousands of man-made chemical compounds that we see today. So our genes have problems to accept these chemicals and respond normally to them as any normal, nonallergic person would do towards chemicals.

Our genes have the innate ability to get adapted to new environments, substances or life-styles. If genes are permitted to live in healthy conditions and surroundings they will likely get adapted to new environments naturally and smoothly, without creating havoc. This may be the reason why people who are born to healthy parents, and live in clean and healthy environments have greater health. People may be sick for the rest of their lives when they: are born to unhealthy, or abusive, parents; are exposed to toxic chemicals, pesticides, fumes and other toxins in their early days; continue to live in unhealthy conditions; and are victims of physical, physiological or mental abuse in their daily lives. Again, our genes were not properly informed about the kind of mental abuses our present time counterparts suffer in this world. If anyone wishes to live a healthy and happy life, it is mandatory to wake up one's misinformed genes and get them to accept the new products and traumas.

This is where NAET® comes in. NAET® is capable of re-programming the confused brain by erasing wrongly imprinted messages. NAET® can also wake up the part of the genes that was dormant and can re-imprint with correct information about the harmlessness of new chemicals, products or life-styles, so the body can enjoy life and worldly things once again. Some genes are slow learners and some are fast learners. Slow learners may need repeated instruction or introduction to handle each and every item around them. They may need to get many repeated NAET® treatments before they feel they are healthy once again and are confident to live among the toxins. Shortcut NAET® treatments or techniques can harm our bodies or confuse our brains. To be most effective, the NAET® Basic-15 need to be treated one-by-one without going out of the treatment order.

Treating the Basic-15 in the correct order is especially important for chemically sensitive people. These people need to be handled gently. Treating NAET® in the correct order prevents excess stress on their systems, so that their already stressed-out immune system can be calmer and more confident in order to heal back to normalcy.

Chemically sensitive people have very fragile emotional centers in their brains. Every little incident can make these people emotional. Their emotions need constant balancing to allow them to heal completely. NAET® treatments should be designed to balance their emotional health as well.

Today, many people are becoming chemically sensitive, making doctors and patients equally frustrated. Some of these patients live in bubble-like environments. This type of person owns completely confused genes which are likely slow learners. It can take two to three years of continuous treatments with NAET® to reintroduce every item around these people and to replace all incorrect information with accurate messages about the environment. No short cut treatments will work on these people. Again, the good news is this: When chemically sensitive people complete the needed NAET treatments, they too can live normally by enjoying the benefits of the scientific advancements of the 21st Century.

Chemically sensitive patients do not have to spend the rest of their lives in fear or in a bubble anymore. Instead, they too can live like normal people, provided they get treated for their allergies by doctors well trained in NAET®.

I would feel gratified, indeed, if the up-to-date material compiled herein were to contribute to my readers achieving, maintaining and enjoying good health; and if, through readers in the healing profession, an even larger number of people were to receive the possible benefits of NAET®.

I have focused on the issues of chemically sick people in this book "Chemical Sensitivities" to let chemically sensitive people know that they are not alone in this saga of life. I have also tried to inform them of certain means to look into and detect the roots of their problems. Once detected, it will be easier to pull these problems out by their roots. If these people understand their problems, they too can lead normal lives. I have published many books on allergies and NAET®. Most of my books carry descriptions of meridians, and other aspects of energetic therapy. The book, "Say Good-bye to Illness" is the melting pot for health-related information on many areas of health in a very concise form. In the companion books, I focus on particular health issues as each title states, as in "Chemical Sensitivities". This is done to avoid repeated reading of the same material by the previous readers of my books, and to down size each book by cutting down pages with repeated information.

If anyone wishes to learn more about acupuncture meridians and the possible pathological symptoms, or to find out about detailed information on diagnostic testing and evaluations to detect allergies, please read my book "Say Good-bye to Illness". Alternatively, to further enhance your understanding, you may wish to pursue some of the other relevant books and articles listed in the bibliography at the conclusion of this book.

Stay Allergy-Free and Enjoy Better HEALTH!

Devi S. Nambudripad,
M.D., D.C., L.Ac., Ph.D.

Introduction

It is your right to eat whatever food you get or like to eat and digest the food, assimilate it and absorb the essential nutrients from whatever you eat without any trouble. It is also your right to live healthy in whatever environment you live with whomever you live and be happy. If you are able to accomplish this, you can say that you are in a healthy condition. If you are not able to do this you need to have yourself checked out by an NAET® specialist.

People without having any firsthand knowledge of NAET® might get confused by the above statement. On the other hand anyone with some experience with NAET, would agree with me because that is what you can accomplish through NAET®: be healthy and be happy.

People have been suffering from various health disorders for a long time, probably from the beginning of the human existence. No one knows the cause of many disorders. No one really knows the actual cause. Most healthcare practitioners identify disorders according to the signs and symptoms exhibited by the patients. We have symptom-oriented treatments for patients to keep them calm. Symptomatic treatments work very well most of the time. When the symptoms are gone, the doctor is happy, the patients are happy. There are some situations when the symptomatic treatments may not work. Then the doctor is puzzled, patients are confused and disappointed. In today's world this scenario happens very frequently.

NAET® is a non-invasive, drug free, natural solution to eliminate allergies of all types and intensities using a blend of selective energy balancing, testing and treatment procedures from acupuncture/acupressure, allopathy, chiropractic, Kinesiology, and nutritional disciplines of medicine.

NAET® theory believes that some software problems (a virus perhaps?) in your brain-computer is the cause of allergies and allergy-related illnesses.

NAET® is a way to reprogram your brain to its original state. NAET® is the computer virus treatment to help your brain to remove the faulty programs and replace it with the correct ones.

NAET® stresses the importance of life-style changes. Consuming non-allergic foods and drinks, living in a non-allergic environment, using non-allergic materials, associating with non allergic people, getting adequate exercise, maintaining sound mental health, all this means life-style changes. It means giving up eating junk food, eating more nutritious meals and eliminating emotional conflicts and unhappy situations.

NAET® is not a magic cure for anything. It is pure hard work based on stone-hard Oriental medical theory. If you are not willing to work hard, if you expect a magic bullet to cure all your problems instantly, NAET® is not for you. If you are willing to work hard, willing to make changes in your life-style you can get relief of any allergy-based medical symptoms, the ones I have mentioned anywhere in this book or in any of my other books. I have treated every one of those allergy-based problems successfully with NAET®. If the patient's presenting problems are not due to allergies then NAET is not the way to treat your problems.

The main application of NAET® is to remove the adverse reactions between your body and other substances around you and thus to provide your body with good nutrition, and enhance the natural ability to absorb, assimilate the necessary elements from the food and eliminate the unwanted and toxic materials when they get into the body by any means. NAET advises you to test everything around you for possible allergy before you use anything new or consume a new food. If you are allergic to every ingredient in the diet, no matter how pure and clean the diet is, you will never feel healthy. Now you can detect if the item is good for you or not before you use or consume them. If the item is not good for you, you do not have to use that particular item, but you can get a substitute.

When you get treated for the known allergens with NAET®, you will not react to these allergens anymore with the future contacts. When you get them into the body, if the items are not useful to the body, body will throw them out through natural elimination process without creating havoc in the immune system.

With this book you can now understand how allergies affect you and produce illnesses mimicking severe health disorders. You may need to go to an NAET® practitioner for several sessions or do it yourself if you have only mild or hidden allergies. When you read this book, you will learn how allergies and allergy-related illness can now be controlled.

NAET® was developed by Dr. Devi S. Nambudripad, who has been treating patients with this technique since 1983, and teaching other health professionals how to administer it since 1989. To date, more than 8,500 licensed medical practitioners and over

150 veterinary doctors have been trained in NAET® procedures and are practicing all over the world. For more information on NAET® or for an NAET® practitioner near you, log on to the NAET® website: www.naet.com.

How Do I Know I Have Allergies?

If you experience any unusual physical, physiological or emotional symptoms without any obvious reason, you can suspect an allergy.

Who Should Use this Book?

Anyone who is suffering from allergies or allergy-related health disease or condition should read this book. This natural, non invasive technique is ideal to treat infants, children, grown-ups, old and debilitated people who suffer from mild to severe allergic reactions without altering their current plan of treatment. NAET encourages the use of all medications, supplements or other therapies while going through the NAET program. When the patient gets better, the patient's regular physician can reduce or alter the dosage of drugs.

How is this Book Organized?

Chapter 1-Explains chemical sensitivities in general terms.

Chapter 2-Describes categories of allergens

Chapter 3- Explains Nambudripad's Testing Techniques and gives you information on various other allergy testing techniques.

Chapter 4- Describes normal and abnormal functions of acupuncture meridians.

Chapter 5-Explains NST(NeuroMuscular Sensitivity testing) to detect allergies.

Chapter 6-Discusses a few of the self-testing and home-self-treatment procedures.

Chapter 7-A collection of NAET Cases and testimonials are given here.

Glossary- This section will help you to understand the appropriate meaning of the medical terminology used in this book.

Resources-Provided to assist you in finding natural products and consultants to support you while you work with your allergies.

Bibliography- Since NAET is an energy balancing treatment, supporting bibliography on this subject is hard to find. This book cannot be completed without mentioning valuable information on Oriental Medicine and acupuncture, because NAET was developed from Oriental Medicine. Since NAET uses basic information from allopathy, kinesiology and chiropractic, books explaining these subject are also given in the bibliography.

Index- A detailed index is included to help you locate your area of interest quickly and easily.

HELPFUL SUGGESTIONS TO THE PROSPECTIVE NAET® PATIENT

I. Introduction

The prospective NAET® patient is required to read Say Good-bye to Illness or Say Good-bye to Your Allergies before coming for the first treatment. NAET® is a method that helps to balance energies in the body. According to Oriental medical theory, when one's body energies are maintained in a balanced state, one does not suffer from most health disorders that arise from an energy imbalance. According to NAET® theory, allergies cause energy imbalances in the energy meridians, also known as energy pathways. An energy blockage is the primary cause for any allergic reaction towards any substance. When the energy blockage from an allergen is removed via NAET®, that particular allergen has not been shown to produce adverse reactions in the body on future contacts. NAET® is a mild, energy balancing, noninvasive, gentle procedure. It has not been shown to cause any long-term adverse effects on anyone within the last twenty years. While going through NAET® treatments, patients should try to keep their symptoms under control by taking necessary medications, therapies or other modalities. The patient is required to seek care of a primary care physician while getting NAET® treatment. If you suffer from a specific problem, you should also seek care of an appropriate medical specialist to manage health needs related to your condition. NAET® is only an energy-blockage removal treatment. NAET® is not a primary care procedure.

II. Before the First Treatment

1. When you arrive at the office, these guidelines will be provided to you or your guardian or caretaker. You (they) MUST read and comply with these rules before beginning the testing procedures.

2. You should bring in a copy of ALL previous medical records, laboratory and radiological reports. You will be required to complete the following forms in the office: Personal data information sheet, history forms, symptom-survey form, and a consent form.

3. If you have a history of anaphylactic reactions toward any allergen, you must tell the NAET® practitioner before beginning the tests. Doing so, your NAET® practitioner can take adequate precaution to prevent you from becoming anaphylactic during treatments.

4. If you have a history of ANAPHYLAXIS, you should inform your practitioner on the very first visit before beginning the testing and treatments. People with history of anaphylaxis should ALWAYS be treated through a surrogate. They should wash their hands or rub both hands together immediately after each treatment. If you have severe allergies or anaphylactic history on any basic group of allergens, (Egg, milk, wheat, fish, etc.) those allergens should be treated after completing rest of the Basic Fifteen groups. People with anaphylaxis are not required to hold the sample during the 20-minute waiting period.

5. NAET® Anaphylactic protocol SHOULD be followed strictly while getting treated. Your NAET® practitioner will instruct you appropriately.

III. Before Each Treatment

6. PLEASE do not wear any perfume, perfumed powder, strong smelling deodorant, hair spray, or after-shave and do not eat strong smelling herbs like raw garlic, seafood, etc., when coming to the NAET® clinic for treatments. If you suspect something is responsible for causing an allergic reaction, you may bring the item to the NAET® office in a thin glass container with a lid (as in a baby food jar with lid), wrapped in brown paper or a brown paper bag. Please

do not bring items in plastic containers. Plastic containers cannot be used in testing.

7. There is NO smoking allowed in or around the office. PLEASE take a shower before you come for a treatment, and wear clean clothes to avoid smells of herbs, spices, perspiration, etc. Various smells can cause irritation and reactions in other sensitive patients in the clinic waiting room. Please do not eat or drink in the office. Another patient in the office waiting room might react to the smell of your food.

8. Wear minimum or no jewelry when you come in for a treatment. Avoid wearing large crystals or large diamonds. NAET® can be done while wearing your own clothes provided you wear simple, loose clothes without ANY art work or embroidery with crystals, beads, stones, metals, glass or plastic pieces. It is fine to wear simple wrist watches while testing or treatments. Avoid watches with sharp needles, cell phones, calculators, tape recorders, photo camera, etc.

9. PLEASE do not wear any guns or knives to the office even when they are part of your job requirements. Please do NOT bring sharp metal objects, large keys, sharp toys, heavy toys, or toy guns to the office.

10. Please turn off your cell phones inside the waiting room and in the treatment room. Other sensitive patients might react to your cell phone. Cell phones should be off and kept away from your body during NAET® testing and desensitization treatment.

11. ALWAYS eat before you come for the treatment. You should not take NAET® treatments and acupuncture when you are hungry. If you have a long wait in your practitioner's office, please bring a snack with you, leave it in the car or outside the office. Five to ten minutes before your treatment, please go outside the clinic and eat your food, wash your hands with soap and water, and rinse your mouth before you return to the clinic for the treatment.

12. Please WASH your hands with soap and water before beginning the Neuromuscular sensitivity testing procedure (NST). Handwashing will remove any residue left on your hands from other substances.

13. Do NOT treat with NAET® if you are extremely tired, worked a night shift, or worked too many hours without a break.

IV. During Each Treatment

14. You should NOT have any companion with you standing or sitting within your magnetic field during treatment. You should not bring any children or pets to the treatment room while you are being treated. You should be alone with your NAET® practitioner while you get tested or treated with NAET®.

15. Since NAET® is a mind-body balancing procedure, the NAET® practitioner needs to receive permission from your conscious and subconscious minds before performing any energy balancing procedures. Signing the consent is the permission from the conscious mind. But permission from the subconscious is necessary for a successful NAET treatment. For a trained practitioner it takes only a few seconds to seek permission from the subconscious. In rare occasions, it has been shown that certain person's subconscious mind does not grant permission to perform NAET® testing or treatment. In such cases, the NAET® practitioner may NOT proceed with NAET® testing. Instead the NAET® practitioner will make appropriate referrals for further evaluations related to their health conditions.

16. The NAET® practitioner must get permission from YOUR subconscious mind before each NAET® desensitization treatment as well. On a particular visit, if your brain did not give favorable signals for a new treatment, you will be rescheduled for another date.

Freedom From Chemical Sensitivities

This is for your best benefit. It has been shown that even anaphylactic cases also can be treated successfully for the anaphylaxis-producing allergen when the NAET® practitioner gets permission from the patient's brain before doing the treatment. You may rest for a few days until your brain and body are ready to get more treatments or you may be able to receive other immune system supporting treatments like chiropractic adjustments, acupuncture, massage, Yoga, etc. while waiting.

17. While performing NST, the patient SHOULD wash or rub his/her hands together for 30 seconds between touching different samples. The energy of the previously tested sample has shown to produce false results if the energy of the previous item has not been removed from the hands before touching a new one.

18. While receiving NST testing or NAET® desensitization procedures PLEASE make a loose fist with your free hand (one without the allergen) in order to prevent contact between the table or your clothes with your fingers while testing.

19. Do not eat or chew gum or candy DURING NST testing or NAET® treatment.

20. The NAET® practitioner will not have ANYONE observing the treatment or taking notes, from a close proximity. The distance varies with each patient for each allergen. Your practitioner will know how to determine the distance.

21. If you are unable to test yourself (if you are a child, old person, too strong, too weak, disabled, advanced stage of pregnancy, etc.), then you SHOULD be tested through a surrogate so that the practitioner can get accurate information about your sensitivities. You should maintain skin-to-skin contact with the surrogate during testing and the surrogate should rub his/her hands together or wash hands between testing different allergens.

22. You could also be treated through a surrogate's body and get the exact benefit as if you were getting treated directly. Patients in advanced stage of pregnancy, morbidly obese, with psoriasis or other debilitating skin problem, back surgery, scoliosis, or a history of anaphylaxis, etc., SHOULD receive NAET® treatments through a surrogate.

V. The Basic 15 treatments

23. The NAET Basic 15 treatments are in fact the basic essential nutrients for everyone. If you are allergic to them your body may not receive adequate nutrients. That will cause to lower the immune system function and may cause to have various health disorders due to nutritional deficiencies brought on by allergies. When your immune system is maintained at a normal level, not only you feel better overall, your allergic sensitivity will be reduced with the result, you need fewer NAET® treatments to get maximum results.

VI. Reasons Why Treatments May Need to be Given Out of Order

24. If you have allergies to white rice, or pasta, they can be treated before the Basic treatments.

25. Hard-to-avoid items like prescription drugs should be treated first in the doctor's office, then treated at home through self-treatment every two hours. In case of a drug that cannot be avoided, you should treat by gate-massage before and after you take the drug as well as massaging the gates every two hours for the 25 hours after the initial treatment.

26. When a patient has an ACUTE problem, practitioners will treat the acute problem before resuming the normal order of treatments if the patient's brain gives permission to do so. For instance, when a patient is reacting to a particular food that was eaten recently, a

medication that is essential for the patient's survival (like pain medication, cortisone, antihistamine, antidepressants, heart medication, etc.), fire-smoke, accidental exposure to fumes, drinking water, city water, acute emotional imbalances like the death of a loved one, etc., can be treated as an acute allergen before completing the basic fifteen treatments as long as the body permits. If someone has severe reaction to pollens, weeds, cigarette smoke, regular drugs like chemotherapy drugs, antibiotics, standard emotional blockage removal treatments, person-to-person allergies, etc., can be treated after completing six basic treatments (after completing sugar mix). When the treatment for acute allergen is completed satisfactorily, you should go back to the basics and continue as before.

VII. After Treatments

27. You must wash your hands with plain water after treatment BEFORE you leave the office. After the treatment if you cannot wash or rinse your hands, vigorously rubbing your hands by interlacing your fingers for 30 seconds will be sufficient.

28. After the NAET® desensitization, PLEASE do not exercise vigorously for 6 hours. A mild walk is fine.

29. AVOID exposure to extreme hot or cold temperature after the desensitization treatment.

30. Do NOT bathe or shower for 6 hours following the NAET® treatment.

31. Do not read or touch other objects with your FINGERS during the 20 minutes waiting period after NAET® treatment.

32. Do NOT cross your hands or feet during the first 20 minutes following the NAET® treatment. Lying or resting with a calm mind will be beneficial. You could visualize positive, warm energy circu-

lation through the 12 meridians while resting. Meditation is allowed. After an emotional NAET®, you are advised to think positively during the 20 minute waiting period about the issue which was treated.

33. Your practitioner WILL ask you to avoid the treated allergen for 25 hours or more as indicated by his/her testing after the completion of the treatment in the office. After the treatment you should avoid eating, touching, breathing and coming within 5 feet of the substance that was treated following 25 hours after treatment. It is also suggested after completing your treatment satisfactorily for an allergen, that you consume a small amount of the item daily for three to four days. If the treatment is not completely finished, you will bring out some minor symptoms and your practitioner can investigate the reasons behind those symptoms and eliminate them. Another benefit of introducing the treated allergen into your body is to reconfirm the brain and nervous system about the harmlessness of the item so that your nervous system will not forget about this allergen in the future even if you never ate them later for years.

34. It is highly recommended that after three NAET® basic treatments, you TRY to consume foods and drinks from the desensitized groups only. Add new items to your list as you complete each treatment. This will reduce your overall discomfort while going through the rest of the treatments and your NAET® treatments will be more effective and you will be able to see results with NAET® faster. Depending on your immune system the treatments can be scheduled. A patient with severe allergies and poor immune system can only tolerate one treatment per week. But patients with better immune system have shown to tolerate three or more treatments per week. Your practitioner can test your body for the appropriate treatment plan.

35. If you are a highly SENSITIVE person, or if you experience any discomfort during the 25 hour-avoidance period after the treat-

ment (crying spells, depression, unusual emotions or unusual pains anywhere in the body, etc.), you may need to balance your gates every two hours on your own at home while you are AWAKE. When you sleep, you do not need to set an alarm to wake you every two hours. Instead whenever you wake up, you can continue treating again.

36. The practitioner can determine the APPROXIMATE number of hours of avoidance by using question response testing for patients who have difficulty avoiding food for 25 hours. Infants and children can be treated in the evening or before going to sleep for hard-to-avoid items. Please ask your practitioner if you have questions.

37. If someone has a hard time avoiding the allergen for a specific amount of time for any particular reason, he/she should BALANCE his/her gate points every two hours as well as before and after exposure to the allergen. In case the patient has developmental disabilities, caretakers should be instructed to massage the gate points (Read Page 58 in the book, Living Pain Free by the author) every two hours during the 25 hours and also before and after touching the treated allergen. Your practitioner will teach you the self-balancing technique if you do not understand by reading the book, Living Pain Free. It is advisable for you to BUY this self-help book with Illustrations since it can help you to control or reduce various allergic reactions and discomforts arising from untreated allergies by massaging the appropriate acupressure self-treatment points whenever the need arises.

38. No adverse reactions have been noted when a person eats food INCLUDING the food he/she was treated, for 20 minutes following the retest of the initial treatment for the allergen. The 25 hour-restriction begins 30 minutes after the completion of the treatment. Do not eat HEAVY meals before or after the NAET® or acupuncture treatments, but DRINK a glass of water before the NAET® treatment. Energy moves better in a well hydrated body.

Drink 4-6 glasses of water through the day after NAET® treatments to help flush out the toxins produced during the treatment.

39. You are advised to MAINTAIN your own treatment and food diary in The Guide Book after each treatment. Write down all the good and bad symptoms you experience during 25-hours following treatment and bring it to your practitioner on your next visit. If you have frequent health problems and you do not know the cause of your problems, write down your daily activities for a month in a separate notebook. Record all the food and drinks you consumed even if they were in small portions and record also anything new you have purchased in the house or work area since the problem started. Bring your record to the office and let your NAET® practitioner test you for the items in your list to find the culprit.

40. You may need to take EXTRA precaution while you get treated for environmental substances: (mineral mix, metals, water, leather, formaldehyde, fabric, wood, mold, mercury, newspaper, chemicals, flowers, etc.). Apart from staying away from these items, you may also need to wear a mask, gloves, socks, shoes, gowns, scarves, earplugs, etc. You can also massage the gate points every two hours while awake during the 25-hour period if it is not completely avoidable.

41. During the 25-hours or afterwards, if you get a life-threatening reaction from an allergen (either from the one you were treated in the office or another one), you MUST seek emergency help immediately from a primary care physician or emergency room, or by calling 911.

42. Once every month or so, or after completing treatments for TEN to FIFTEEN allergens, your practitioner will repeat NST on all treated allergens. If an allergen wasn't passing over 50 percent at the time, they will be boosted up again. No avoidance is necessary at this time.

43. AFTER the Basic Fifteen treatments with the practitioner, patient should begin to gather a small sample of every day food and drinks and holding the sample, balance the gate points every night before bedtime.

44. DRINK one 6 ounce-glass of water first thing in the morning. Drink 1 glass of water before bedtime.

45. Remember to CHECK with your practitioner for the item you treated, after 25 hours, and at least within one week to make sure you have completed the treatment.

VII. Additional Information about NAET®

46. NAET® is a HOLISTIC procedure. It balances the entire body including: physical, physiological and emotional functions. Everyone needs balance in all these levels of the body to be healthy. If one area is not balanced properly, other areas cannot function normally. NAET® emotional balancing procedure has been shown to produce marvelous results in people who suffer from environmental illness, chemical reactions, chronic pain disorders, other chronic illnesses, autism and ADHD, etc. This emotional balancing treatment will be provided to the patient without additional cost if done in conjunction with a treatment for another substance. After completion of Sugar treatment (after completing six basic treatments), NAET® emotional balancing treatments can be administered upon request.

47. NAET® emotional balancing procedures do NOT replace the need for traditional psychological or psychiatric help. If you are getting treatments in these areas prior to NAET®, please continue with your therapies and medications as needed. If you for any reason do not like to be balanced emotionally by your NAET® practitioner (due to religious reasons, etc.), you should inform the

NAET® practitioner on the initial visit, then emotional balancing procedure will be excluded from your treatment plan.

48 If you did not complete the treatment, or if you could not complete the specific NAET® treatment for some reason, do not panic. NAET® is a mild, energy balancing, noninvasive, gentle procedure. It has not been shown to cause any long-term adverse effects on anyone since its discovery within the last twenty-three years. Your temporary symptoms may be due to the incomplete treatment and may continue for up to two or three weeks maximum. Drink about 4-6 glasses of boiled cooled water daily to help with your energy circulation.

49. Eventually the particular symptoms will wear off and you may return to your pre-NAET® status if you did not repeat the treatment for the unfinished allergen. For example, if you suffered from insomnia prior to NAET® treatment, you may continue to have insomnia; if you suffered from pain disorders, you may continue to suffer from pain disorders, etc. An allergen which was treated halfway has not shown to render any benefit to the patient at all. Human body forgets and adapts to new ways fast. The incomplete treatment is forgotten in about three days to a week in most cases, but in some cases it has shown to take as long as three weeks, then the body learns to focus on current events. Thus, in a few days, an incompletely treated allergen is usually viewed by the body as an allergen that has never been treated before.

50. But if you had to stop the NAET treatment for the particular allergen because you had no means to get to the office, then you can balance the energy for the particular item at home on your own by holding the item while massaging the gate points once every four hours while awake for two to three weeks or as short or as long as the body needs to view that as a friendly item. This method will only work after one has been treated initially with a trained practitioner, and the treatment was not completed for some reason. If it is an uncomplicated, individual item, like a piece of

sourdough bread, a piece of meat, a hot dog, a laxative or a pain pill like Tylenol or another drug, a particular piece of fabric (a shirt, scarf), etc., then the patient or the caretaker can complete the treatment in this manner at home. CAUTION: this should be done only on a single allergen, never try on a group of allergens.

51. After completing treatment for an allergen, if NST tested strong on retest but the patient is still suffering from prior symptoms, the patient should be allowed to rest a few days to a couple of weeks without any new NAET® treatment. This is in fact to rule out or to determine if the desensitization towards the particular allergen was successful or not; and to determine if the presenting symptom is arising from another source or not. If the particular allergen treatment is incomplete, if you wait a few days the NST will produce a weak response either on its own or with some combinations. Then the treatment on the allergen itself or with a combination can be repeated at that time. While waiting to detect the outcome of the previous treatment, it is OK to boost up the immune system with acupuncture, chiropractic treatments, massages, herbs or other therapies. Or the patient can continue to self balance for the item at home as described above.

52. Sometimes, the patient continues to have the same symptom but NST does not show any weakness on the previously treated allergen. In such cases it has shown that the patient passed the treated allergen but another allergen capable of producing similar symptoms has been identified as the culprit. Usually people with history of allergies react to more than one or a few allergens. When one allergen gets desensitized and eliminated from the body, others will get noticed easier, hence the symptom of the previous allergen continues until all the allergens are desensitized with NAET®.

53. When one has a weakness in any particular area of the body, every allergen affects that area of the body giving rise to symptom similar to the first one. This pattern is especially noticed in patients with asthma, sinus problems, autistic disorders, attention-deficit

hyperactive disorders, chronic pain syndrome, as in degenerative arthritis, fibromyalgia, lupus, headaches, migraines, backaches, myofascial pain, peripheral neuropathy, PMS, insomnia, manic or depressive disorders, etc. Because of this mechanism, until you complete NAET® for Basic Fifteen, you may not see much changes in your health in these cases.

54. When you are allergic to a substance, your body produces lots of endogenous toxins. After you are treated to an allergen, it takes 24 hours for the body to detoxify the allergen from all 12 major meridians (each meridian takes 2 hours) naturally to get the toxins out of the body. SOME patients may not have 24 hour avoidance or restrictions. Some may pass the allergen right after the treatment; some may take just a few hours; some may take 25 hours, yet some others may take 40 hours. Even though NST demonstrated that you would clear the allergen in 10 minutes or so, it is to your advantage to avoid the item for the whole 25 hours (24 hours plus one hour guard-band) allowing the body to detox naturally. After a few NAET® treatments, you have the option to go on a good detoxification program using different products (herbs, minerals, etc.) to clean up your system. But if you faithfully follow the 25-hour avoidance, you may not need any special detoxification since the body is able to naturally eliminate the toxins in time if given a chance.

55. You are advised to continue ALL medications and other treatment modalities as they have been prescribed unless otherwise directed by the doctors who prescribed them. PLEASE do not stop any other treatment you are on: medication, therapy, chiropractic treatments, massages, etc.

56. NAET® treatments have NOT been shown to interfere with any other treatment. In fact, if you can keep your body free of toxin accumulation and keep your symptoms under control by using medication or therapies, NAET® has shown to work better.

57. For FEMALE patients: Treatments are not advisable during the first three days of menstrual cycle.

58. NAET® treatments during pregnancy have not shown to cause any adverse effects to the mother or child so far. In fact tremendous benefits have been noted in both cases. When the mothers receive adequate NAET® treatments during pregnancy (at least 15 basics and all known allergens of the mother treated), their children are born with very few allergies when compared with their siblings who never had exposure to NAET® before birth.

59. When you go through the NAET® treatment program, you will be advised to get supplemented with appropriate amount of vitamins, minerals, and other nutrients for a while if it is indicated. When the nutrients are supplemented appropriately pain and discomfort arising from various disorders like chronic fatigue, general body aches, arthritis, and other pain disorders due to deficiencies, etc., will be reduced.

60. If you do not show any improvement in your health status after successfully passing Basic ten to fifteen allergen groups at all three levels, probably NAET® is not for you. Please ask your practitioner to refer you to another source of healthcare facility.

Signature of the patient/guardian _____

Date_____

Print Your name _____

Witness _____

1

MSG Sensitivity

Dear Devi:

This letter is for you, Mala, Mohan, Kris, and Janna. Beginning in 1971, I began to have periods of disorientation, inability to "find" words when I spoke, unstable walk pattern, and facial rash. On some occasions, I went into anaphylactic shock, with a precipitous drop in blood pressure. The diagnosis made by several physicians was MSG-sensitivity.

For some time, I was able to protect myself by avoiding the food ingredient monosodium glutamate. However, as the food industry began to use more and more ingredients that included the reactive component of monosodium glutamate, (processed free glutamic acid), I very often experienced a feeling of not feeling well, and, from time to time, had more bouts of anaphylaxis. I have lost consciousness more than 30 times since 1971.

As my tolerance for all processed free glutamic acid (MSG) became lower and lower, I had more difficulty staying well. I began to limit my eating to home prepared meals. In fact, if I had to be away from home for more than a few hours, I carried food with me. I did not even risk eating at my children's homes. My reactions began to include periods of atrial fibrillation following MSG ingestion.

At the time that I learned about NAET®, I was having difficulty eating safely, even though I only ate meals that I had prepared. At this point, the glutamate and food industry was using processed free glutamic acid (MSG) in most processed foods, and farmers had begun to spray some crops with a pesticide that included processed free glutamic acid (MSG). At this point, I even lost consciousness from a plain baked potato. During a 60 day period, I experienced a number of episodes of atrial fibrillation, and was debilitated 44 out of the 60 days recorded.

As an individual who spent my entire life working in and with allopathic medical facilities, I had great concern about trying NAET®, but felt that I could not continue living as I was. You may recall, I only agreed to start NAET® after meeting with you and getting answers to a number of questions that I had. During testing, Mohan noted that one of the diagnostic procedures that you use indicated that I had a very low energy level.

I now have completed the NAET® treatments that appear to apply to my condition. I have decided to try to go on at this point without further treatment, knowing that if I have problems, all of you will be there to help me. I now feel better than I have in many years, in spite of the fact that I will soon be 68 years old. I now can again eat without fear at my children's homes, go to the homes of friends for dinner, travel, and eat out in restaurants. In short, NAET® has given me my life back.

I have spent many years in the health care industry. During those years, I have never met anyone more kind and dedicated to helping people than you, Mala, Mohan, and Kris. The good feelings about your office begin with the greeting by Janna when one enters your office.

I can understand that some people in the health care industry who have not had the misfortune of having food and environmental allergies and/or sensitivities, and who have not experienced the "miracles" that can be realized through NAET® treatments, may express concern about NAET®, but, as former NAET® patients know, NAET® does work. Although it appears that more people are learning about the value of NAET®, I wish it were used even more broadly by health care practitioners than it is, including by allopathic physicians.

I do not know how to thank all of you at the office for allowing me to enjoy the balance of my life. I will miss seeing all of you weekly at the office, but will stop in from time to time to let you know how I am doing. Thank you Devi for having the courage to offer NAET® to patients in need, knowing that NAET® would be controversial in the minds of some.

Sincerely yours,
Jack L. Samuels

CAUSES OF CHEMICAL SENSITIVITIES

Disruption of the software program of the brain: The main cause of allergies and sensitivities is the computer software error in one's brain-computer or let's say one's brain-computer software has a 'Virus.' This virus causes malfunction of the software, in turn all body functions are disrupted. This causes the body to be sensitive to everything around the body, especially to all chemicals. The malfunctioning program does not recognize the man-made chemicals around the body anymore. This software virus may have found its way into the body through the following routes:

• Heredity: An allergic tendency towards chemicals is inherited from parents and family as dominant or recessive, but allergic manifestation may vary from generation to generation. For example, if a parent suffered from migraines whenever she ate chocolate, offspring may suffer from eczema or asthma whenever he/she smelt coffee or ate chocolate and not necessarily have migraines when exposed to caffeine products.

• Toxins: From food, drinks, medicines, herbs, vitamins, environments, animal epithelial, animal dander, pesticides, lead, mercury, dry cleaning chemicals, house cleaning chemicals, chemically treated city water, drinking water, industrial waste, polluted air, automobile exhaust, carbon monoxide, pollen, smoke, cigarette smoke, etc.

• Infections: Toxins produced in the body from invasions of microorganisms such as virus, bacteria, parasite, yeast, candida, ticks (lyme disease), etc.

- Vaccinations and immunizations and toxins produced by the interaction of the body with these drugs.

- A depressed immune system: Chronic illnesses, autoimmune disorders, etc.

- Malabsorption disorders: Nutritional deficiencies, digestive problems, poor absorption and assimilation of nutrients due to an allergy to the nutrients, eating overcooked, contaminated, or unsuitable food or unavailability of nutritious food. Many people are sensitive to foods cooked in microwave ovens.

- Hormonal deficiencies: Removal of reproductive organs, dysfunction of ovaries, thyroid glands, hypothalamus, deficiency of female and male hormones, adrenals and pituitary hormones.

- Posttraumatic disorders: Surgery, accidents, delivery, stressful work, school, life-style, war veterans, etc.

- Radiation and geopathic stress: Working long hours with computers, sitting in front of television sets, living near or under powerful electrical cables, living near power plants, exposure to radioactive materials, working under extreme weather conditions without proper clothing.

- Poor Physical Activities

- Emotional traumas: Disharmony of mind-body-spirit due to traumas from past or present, childhood abuses, abuses and traumas at other ages, troubled emotions like chronic fear, anger, cult association, victimization, etc. Another source for chronic illnesses is emotional involvement from past generations and the emotional effect (fear, helplessness, etc.) is transferred into people through genes. We have documented several such cases in whom dramatic health improvements were noted after clearing through NAET® the effects of emotionally fearful incidents that happened to their ancestors.

In people with allergies, the normal imprint (memory) about the harmlessness of substances such as peanut, fish, pollen, dust, perfume, etc., has somehow been erased from the brain's memory during the genetic transference or during certain stresses of life (exposure to extreme radiation, bacterial or chemical toxins, genetic mutation, etc.) and has substituted the memory with new information that identifies the substance as being dangerous. Thus, the immune system mistakes a harmless substance for a dangerous intruder it must destroy. When a person with allergies is exposed to something it perceives to be an allergen, the immune system produces antibodies to fight it as a harmful invader.

Allergies usually first appear in infancy or childhood. However, onset of symptoms can occur at any age or, in some cases, reappear after many years of inactivity. An allergy is generally a hereditary condition. An allergic tendency is inherited, but it may manifest totally differently than that of one's ancestors. The age of onset of an allergic condition depends on the degree of inheritance. The stronger the genetic factor, the earlier in life is the onset. Studies have shown that when both parents were (or are) allergy-sensitive, 75 to 100 percent of their offspring react to the same or similar allergens. When neither of the parents is (or was) sensitive to allergens, the probability of producing allergic offspring drops dramatically, to less than ten percent.

The actual fact is that there are hardly any human diseases or conditions in which allergic factors are not involved either directly or indirectly. Any substance under the sun, including sunlight itself, can cause an allergic reaction in any individual.

In other words, potentially, you can be allergic to anything you come in contact with. If you begin to check people around you—even so-called healthy people—you will find hidden allergies as a causative factor in almost all health problems.

For those whose lives are merely disrupted by the discomfort of the reaction, traditional treatments with simple antihistamine or topical remedies can bring relief. But for more serious sufferers, either long-term immunotherapy or complete avoidance is the only hope traditional medicine has generally been able to offer. Immunotherapy, of course, is very expensive and time consuming, and it often does not present a satisfactory outcome. Most people finally resort to a lifetime of depriving themselves of the many things in life that would otherwise bring them joy and fulfillment. Common complaints are, *"My allergies have taken control of my life,"* and *"The very things that I want to make me happy are the very things that I react to the most."*

Even with avoidance, there is no guarantee that allergy sufferers will be able to stay away from every situation and still remain reaction free. With the progress of science and technology, our modern life-styles have changed dramatically. New products, which are potential allergens for many people, are being developed every day. The quality of life has improved; but for some allergic patients, the scientific achievements have created more nightmares.

We cannot ignore the fact that we are in the twenty-first century where technology is ever more predominant than before. There is nothing wrong with the technology. In fact, modern technology has provided a better quality of life. But the allergic patient must find ways to overcome adverse reactions to chemicals and other allergens produced by the technology in order to enjoy living in this world.

Even though it requires a series of detailed treatments, NAET® offers the prospect of relief to those who suffer from constant allergic reactions by reprogramming the brain to perfect health. Just like rebooting a computer, we can reboot our nervous system through NAET®and overcome the adverse reactions of brain and body and the person can resume living a normal life.

To comprehend NAET® and chemical sensitivity, some understanding of the brain and its functions is necessary. Many books on the subject of the brain are available in bookstores and libraries. A brief introduction to brain functioning related to NAET® is given here. For more information, please consult the references in the bibliography.

THE BRAIN AND THE NERVOUS SYSTEM

Study of the nervous system is a complex subject even to students of the neurological sciences. I do not expect every reader to comprehend all the material presented below on the nervous system and its functions. To understand the nervous system, one must know its organization, the mechanism of communication and the signaling pathways. Then it will be easier to comprehend the relationship between the nervous system, the immune response (one of the main functions of the nervous system) and the treatment that has been found extremely useful in regulating the function of the nervous system and the immune response. This treatment is known as NAET® or Nambudripad's Allergy Elimination Techniques.

ORGANIZATION

The nervous system is comprised of the central nervous system and the peripheral nervous system. The spinal cord and brain are the two components of the central nervous system.

THE BRAIN

The brain can be divided into six major parts:

1. Medulla
2. Pons
3. Cerebellum
4. Midbrain/Thalamus
5. Cerebral hemispheres
6. Cerebral Cortex

The brain is the master control center of the body and constantly receives information from the sensory nerve fibers about conditions both inside and outside the body. It rapidly analyzes this information and then sends out messages that control body functions, actions and reactions (responses). It also stores all information from past experiences that happened in or around the body at three levels (physical, physiological and emotional), which makes learning and remembering possible. In addition, the brain is the source of thoughts, moods and emotions.

THE NERVOUS SYSTEM

Before the invention of the compound microscope, nervous tissue was thought to function like a gland. In the beginning of the first century, Greek physician Galen proposed that nerves circulate a special kind of fluid secreted by the brain and spinal cord to the body's periphery. In the eighteenth century, the microscope revealed the true structure of the cells of the nervous tissue. Even so, nervous tissue did not become the subject of a special science until the late 1800's, when the first detailed descriptions of nerve cells were undertaken by Camillo Golgi and Santiago Ramon Y Cajal.

Golgi was able to view the neuron under the microscope. He was able to see that neurons had cell bodies and two major projections, a branching dendrite at one end and a long cable-like axon at the other. Ramon Y Cajal was able to stain individual cells, thus showing that nervous tissue is not one continuous web, but a network of discrete cells. In the course of this work, Ramon Y Cajal developed some of the key concepts and much of the early evidence for the principle that individual neurons are the elementary signaling elements of the nervous system.

Physiological investigation of the nervous system began in the late 1700's when the Italian physician and physicist Luigi Galvani discovered that living, excitable muscle and nerve cells produced electricity. Modern electrophysiology grew out of work in the 19th century by three German physiologists—Emil Du Bois-Reymond, Johannes Muller, and Hermann Von Helmholtz—who were able to show that the electrical activity of one nerve cell affects the activity of an adjacent cell in predictable ways.

At the end of the nineteenth century, pharmacology made its first impact on our knowledge of the nervous system and behavior when Claude Bernard in France, Paul Ehrlich in Germany, and John Langley in England demonstrated that drugs do not interact with cells arbitrarily, but rather bind to specific receptors typically located in the membrane on the cell's surface. This discovery became the basis of the all-important study of the chemical basis of communication between nerve cells.

THE BRAIN AND ALLERGIES

The brain works like a computer. Brain cells produce electrical signals and send them from cell to cell along pathways called *circuits*. These electrical circuits receive, process, store, and retrieve information. The brain creates its electrical signals by chemical means.

Sensory information in the central nervous system is processed in stages, in the sequential relay nuclei of the spinal cord, brain stem, thalamus, and cerebral cortex.

The cerebral hemispheres consist of cerebral cortex, basal ganglia, hippocampus and the amygdala.

The basal ganglia helps in regulating motor and sensory activities; the hippocampus participates in storing the memory; and amygdala is involved in coordinating the autonomic and endocrine responses at various levels including emotional level. The cerebral cortex can be further divided into three areas according to their functions:

1. The *sensory cortex* receives messages from the sense organs as well as messages of pressure, pain, and temperature.

2.   The *association cortex* analyzes, processes and stores information about all internal and external stimuli received from the sense organs. Due to this unique functional ability of the association cortex, man is able to display higher mental abilities, such as thinking, speaking, storing, retrieving, correcting and restoring information about everything that happened around him/her.

3.   The *motor cortex* sends out responses to the peripheral nervous system through spinal nerves about the stimuli received from the sense organs. It also controls the movements of all skeletal muscles.

Insult or injury to any cell in these areas is capable of producing abnormal reaction in the associated areas in the body. The proper functioning of the brain depends on many complicated chemical substances produced by the brain cells in these areas.

The spinal cord consists of 31 pairs of spinal nerves. Parasympathetic and sympathetic nerves emerge from the spinal cord and travel to various parts of the body, including body surfaces. There are special sensory receptors seen in certain areas in the peripheral tissue (hands, feet, finger-pads, etc.) These receptors are activated by perceived or actual tissue damage. Harmful stimuli to the skin, subcutaneous tissue or muscle activate the peripheral endings of several classes of sensory receptors, whose cell bodies are located in the dorsal root ganglia. There are certain nerve fibers terminating on neurons in the dorsal horn of the spinal cord, known as afferent nerve fibers. They carry the information further to the thalamus and cerebral cortex.

The synaptic transmission of the information through the nerve fibers is mediated by chemical neurotransmitters, such as neuropeptides, glutamate, serotonin, bradykinin, histamine, prostaglandin, leukotriene, tryptophane, and substance P and more. Neurons in several regions of the cerebral cortex respond selectively to different information arriving at different areas of the cortex. These areas make the appropriate assessment of the incoming stimuli and the responses are relayed back instantly to the specific affected tissue and to the rest of the body via efferent nerve fibers. The arriving messages can produce various sensitivity reactions at the specific sites or in the entire body (hives, itching, redness, sudden fatigue, fainting spells, anger, depression, mania, insecurity, fear, nervousness, etc.)

When there is an insult or injury to the relay centers in the cerebral cortex, the messages do not transmit appropriately through afferent or efferent nerve fibers. During these conditions, the confused chemical mediators take matters into their hands and activate sensory receptors on their own in the pretext of stabilizing the system. Insult to tissue releases chemical messengers such as bradykinin and prostaglandins, which can also activate nociceptors similar to the stimuli arriving from outside the body through the peripheral nervous system. Activation of these sensory receptors (nociceptors) leads to the release of substance P. Substance P acts on mast cells near the sensory nerve endings, causing the release of histamines and other immune system mediators, again hoping to bring the body to a state of homeostasis.

THE COMMUNICATION NETWORK

The central nervous system obtains sensory information from the environment, evaluates the significance of information, and generates appropriate responses. The peripheral nervous system relays information to the central nervous system through the afferent nerves; and when the responses are generated in the brain, the efferent nerves bring them back to the spinal cord and to the peripheral nervous system. The *axon* carries nerve impulses from the cell body to other neurons. The *dendrites* pick up impulses from the axon of other neurons and transmit them to the cell body. The junction where any branch of one neuron transmits a nerve impulse to a branch of another neuron is called a *synapse*. Each neuron may form synapses with thousands of other nerve cells.

NERVE CELLS

Nerve cells are the main signaling units of the nervous system. A typical neuron has four morphologically defined regions: the cell body, dendrites, the axon, and presynaptic terminals. Each of these regions has a distinct role in the generation of signals and the communication of signals between nerve cells.

When the sensory nerve endings (from nasal mucosa, lung, mouth, alimentary tract, skin, fingertips, etc.) gather information about an allergen close to its proximity, it transmits information via afferent nerve fibers to the brain (hypothalamus and to associated parts of the cerebral cortex). The hypothalamus and the parts of the cerebral cortex will relay the information about the allergen's proximity to the rest of the body via electrical signals and alert the entire body. Along with every nerve cell, the body's immune system will be alerted to call upon the defensive forces, with the result the immune response will begin immediately by stimulating lymphocytes to mature into plasma cells, and the plasma cells to produce antibodies (IgE and IgG, etc., suited to the condition) as needed to handle the situation.

The allergens are small antigens that commonly provoke an IgE antibody response. Such antigens normally enter the body at very low doses by diffusion across mucosal surfaces and, therefore, trigger an immune response. The specific IgE produced in response to the allergen binds to the high-affinity receptor for IgE on mast cells, basophils, and activated eosinophils. IgE production can be amplified by these cells. The tendency to IgE over-production is influenced by genetic and environmental factors. Once IgE is produced in response to an allergen, re-exposure to the allergen triggers an allergic response. The allergen triggers the activation of IgE-binding mast cells in the exposed tissue, leading to a series of responses that are characteristic of an allergy.

NAET® INTERVENTION

We propose that NAET intercepts here and puts a stop to the immune response, by deactivating the IgE-binding mast cell function, with the result that the anticipated allergic reaction do not takes place. Not only that, by stimulating the specific afferent and efferent nerves and nociceptors in dorsal root ganglia while the person is in physical contact with the said allergen, the NAET® treatment is able to change the characteristics of the previous stimulus into a new one with a different signal. These altered stimuli will carry new information about the antigen via synapses to the appropriate areas of the cerebral cortex. In return, the brain will relay its response about this new information to every cell in the body. The previously activated immune response will get replaced by this newly relayed signal, causing the erasing and reimprinting of the previously imprinted message about the harmfullness of the substance into one which the nervous system now recognizes as being relatively harmless. This process has been observed in numerous patients to give them an instant, non-allergic response when re-exposed to a substance that was perceived previously as an allergen. NAET® involves the whole brain and its network of nerves as it reprograms the brain by erasing the previous harmful memory regarding the allergen, and imprinting a new, useful memory in its place.

This does not mean that after treating for a harmful chemical, our body does not recognize the chemical as dangerous or harmful. NAET® treatments prepare the brain to respond appropriately to the treated allergen. When the body encounters the treated chemical in the future, the brain (and nervous system) evaluates the energy of the substance. If the energy of the substance is complementary to the body function, it accepts it and if it is not complementary to the body function, the brain releases it without causing panic or turmoil in or around the body.

Someone with no experience with NAET® or who does not understand the complete function of NAET® might ask another question at this time: what if someone who was treated for chlorox (or bleach or any other corrosive chemical) with NAET® and after 25 hours or after clearing the allergy completely decided to drink a glass of the chemical in the morning for breakfast instead of the usual orange juice?

When someone does that we are not talking about the allergy anymore but the dosage and toxicity. NAET® can treat the allergy, it cannot increase your capacity to consume the enormous amounts of the products that you have treated. To test and treat the allergy you need a minute amount of the substance. When you use any product you need to know how much your body can tolerate that substance without causing an overdose problem. It applies not only to the harmful chemicals but to every substance you treated with NAET®. How about foods or drinks? After eliminating the allergy for breads, some people consume endless amount of breads, meats, eggs, just because now they are not allergic to them and the foods taste good. What would be the result? Pack many unwanted pounds in unwanted places in your body. Instead of that if they could only check (using the testing procedures described in Chapter 5 in this book) to see how many slices of bread, how many eggs, how many ounces of meat they could eat comfortably during the course of a day without over-dosing on them, then they could maintain their normal figure for any number of years to come. Using the same principle, one could check to find out how many drops of chlorox one could use a day on his/her body or on the products they use, they would be able to use the treated chemicals without any adverse problem. Anything beyond the body's limit will be seen as an overdose. When one overdoses on food items, one packs pounds on the body because food does not disintegrate the body instantly but chlorox will because that is the action of any corrosive products. So you need to determine how much bleach your body can tolerate without causing toxicity when you decide to drink bleach for breakfast. Probably a drop or two in a glass of water may not cause much toxicity. In fact many studies have shown significant reduction of microflora in the food products (herbs, spices, milk, etc.) when they are washed or preserved with diluted amount of chlorox or bleach or chlorine. Instruction on the preparation of food for emergencies advises to use 16 drops of chlorox per gallon of water or milk. Using sixteen drops of chlorox per gallon of liquid (water or milk) may be OK for someone without any allergy to chlorox. But for someone with an allergy to chlorox this can be hazardous. So please clear the allergy to chlorox before using chlorox for food storage, housecleaning, or washing fabrics or even drinking milk.

Our experience to date has shown that the IgE and IgG antibody levels take a period up to six months or more (in certain cases up to four years) after completing NAET® to drop to lower levels upon retesting for specific antigens. This is quite similar to the findings of traditional allergists that persons who lose reactivity to certain allergens which caused positive Double-Blind Placebo Controlled Food Challenges (DBPCFC's) during childhood will continue to have positive skin tests for these allergens for up to two years after DBPCFC has become negative.

THE EMOTIONAL CONNECTION WITH

ALLERGIES

The emotions we experience involve many areas of the brain as well as other body organs. A part of the brain structure called the *limbic system* plays a central role in the production of emotions. This system consists of parts of the temporal lobe, hypothalamus and thalamus. An emotion may be provoked by a message from a sense organ or by a thought in the cerebral cortex. In either case, nerve impulses are produced and reach the limbic system. These impulses stimulate different areas of the system, depending on the kind of sensory message or thought. For example, the impulses might activate parts of the system that produce pleasant feelings involved in emotions like joy and love. We can easily be inspired and energized by impulses that activate parts of the system that uplift our spirits and bring forth feelings of harmony and well being. These grand moments of reverie are in our power. On the other hand, the impulses that stimulate unpleasant feelings associated with anger and fear can produce negative results.

THE BASIS OF NAET®

A thorough treatise on biochemistry is not appropriate for an introduction to this new method of treatment for people suffering from allergies. Instead, this discussion will concentrate on the basic constructs of the treatment method and give some insight into the lives of the people it has helped.

This is not a new technology. It is actually a combination of knowledge and techniques that uses much of what is already known from allopathic (Western medical knowledge), chiropractic, kinesiology, acupuncture (Oriental medical knowledge) and nutrition. Each of the disciplines I studied provided bits of knowledge which I used in developing this new allergy elimination treatment.

Until now, there has been no known permanent successful method of treatment for chemical sensitivities using Western medicine except avoidance.

I developed this technique of allergy elimination, to identify and treat the reactions to many substances, including food, chemicals, environmental allergens and emotional imbalances caused from allergies.

Through many long years of research, and after many trials and errors, I devised this combination of allergy elimination treatments to eliminate energy blockages (allergies) permanently and to restore the body to a healthy state. These energy blockage elimination techniques together are called *Nambudripad's Allergy Elimination Techniques,* or **NAET®** for short.

WHAT IS NAET®?

NAET® is a non-invasive, drug free, natural solution to eliminate allergies and energy disturbances of all types and intensities using a blend of selective energy balancing, testing and treatment procedures from acupuncture/acupressure, allopathy, chiropractic, Kinesiology, and nutritional disciplines of medicine.

HOW WAS NAET® DISCOVERED?

NAET® was discovered by an accident on Friday, November 23, 1983, at about 2:00 p.m. I was being treated by acupuncture for the relief of a severe allergic reaction to raw carrots. During the treatment, I fell asleep with the carrots still in my hand on my body. After the acupuncture treatment (and a restful nap during the needling period), I woke up and experienced a unique sense of well-being. I had never felt quite that way following other similar acupuncture treatments in the past. I realized that I had been lying on some of the carrot pieces. A piece was also still in my hand. I knew that some of the needles were supposed to help circulate the electrical energy and balance the body. If there is any energy blockage, the balancing process is supposed to clear it during the treatment and bring the body to a balanced state. I had studied this concept in school.

I asked my husband, who was assisting me in the treatment process, to test me for carrots again using NST (Neuromuscular sensitivity Testing explained in detail in Chapter 5). After putting "two and two together," I understood that the carrot's energy field had interacted with my own energy field, and my brain had accepted this once deadly poison to my body as a harmless item now after balancing the two energies during the acupuncture treatment. The two energy fields no longer clashed. This was an amazing NEW DISCOVERY. Subsequent tests for carrots by NST confirmed that something phenomenal had happened. We repeated testing every hour for the rest of that day. I continued eating carrots the next day without any allergic reaction. This confirmed the result. My central nervous system had learned a different response to the stimulus arriving from carrot and I was no longer reactive to it. In some mysterious way, the treatment had reprogrammed my brain.

What followed was a series of experiments treating my own allergies and those of my family. I cured most of my allergies in a year's time. The method was eventually extended to my practice. In every case, allergies were "cleared out," never to return.

After having treated thousands of patients for a wide variety of allergens, the procedure is no longer experimental or of questionable value. It is a proven treatment method and the premise of NAET® methodology that is now being followed by more than 8,500 health-care professionals around the world.

OVERVIEW OF NAET®

Physical contact with the allergen during and after a treatment (which consists of stimulating certain specific points on the acupuncture meridians, thus stimulating the central nervous system) produces the necessary immune mediators or antidotes to neutralize the adverse reaction coming from the allergen held in the hand. This produces a totally new, permanent and irreversible response to the allergen. It is possible, through stimulation of the appropriate points of the acupuncture meridians, (which have direct correspondence with the brain), to reprogram the brain.

A living person's body is made up of bones, flesh, lymph, nerves and blood vessels, which can only function in the presence of vital energy. Like electricity, vital energy is not visible to the human eye.

No one knows how the vital energy gets into the body or how, when or where it goes when it leaves. It is true, however, that without it, none of the body functions can take place. When the body is alive, vital energy flows freely through the energy pathways. Uninterrupted circulation of the vital energy flowing through the energy pathways is necessary to keep the person alive. This circulation of energy makes all the body functions possible. The circulation of the vital energy makes the blood travel through the blood vessels, helping to distribute appropriate nutrients to various parts of the body for its growth, development, functions, and for repair of wear and tear.

The success of the NAET® procedure confirms that a major portion of the illnesses we observe result from allergies.

The evidence suggests a convincing argument can be made that a significant number of patients suffering from latent, undiagnosed allergies, normally treated by traditional Western medical practitioners for temporary relief, are going to experience a cure from NAET® health practitioners without using any invasive therapies. Freedom from allergies is becoming a fact for many patients formerly presenting a wide range of symptoms, from chemical sensitivity and eczema to various types of acute and chronic pain disorders and behavioral problems.

The public should be educated to find the cause of the problems. If the cause can be traced, you can easily avoid contact with the causative agent. If contact is unavoidable, you can go to any of the eighty-five hundred plus NAET® trained medical professionals who have mastered the NAET® method of eliminating the allergy and allergy related problems and get the allergy removed, so that you don't have to avoid the item for ever.

NAET® has its origin in Oriental medicine. Even so, if one explores most Oriental medical books–acupuncture textbooks, one may not find the NAET® interpretation of health problems that I write in my books, because NAET® is my sole development after observing my own reactions, my family's and patients' over the past two decades. Recently, however, information about the effectiveness of NAET® has been given credit in a number of books, but the reader will find correct information of NAET® interpretation of Oriental medical principles only in my books.

In this book, information about acupuncture meridians is kept to a minimum, enough to educate the reader about some traditional functions and dysfunctions of the meridians in the presence of energy disturbances. Some of this information is also available in acupuncture textbooks that one may find in libraries. It is a good idea to have some understanding of Oriental medicine and the meridians when undergoing NAET® treatments although it is not mandatory. To learn more about acupuncture meridians and mind-body connections, please read Chapter 10 in my book *Say Good-bye to Illness.*

NAET® utilizes a variety of standard medical procedures to diagnose and then treat allergies and allergy-related health conditions. These include: standard medical diagnostic procedures and standard allergy testing procedures (read Chapter 3). After detecting allergies, NAET® uses standard chiropractic and acupuncture/acupressure treatments to eliminate them. Various studies have proven that NAET® is capable of erasing the previously encoded incorrect message about an allergen and replacing it with a harmless or useful message by reprogramming the brain. (Please read the Journal of NAET® Energetics and Complementary Medicine, Vol 1, 2, 3 and 4, 2005; Vol 5 and 6, 2006.) This is accomplished by bringing the body into a state of "homeostasis" using various NAET® energy balancing techniques.

Chiropractic theory postulates that a pinching of the spinal nerve root(s) may cause nerve energy disturbance in the energy pathways causing poor nerve energy supply to the target organs (disturbance in the functions of afferent and efferent nerves). When the particular nerve fails to communicate with a particular area of the organs and tissues, normal functions of that area do not take place. The affected organs and tissues then begin to manifest impaired functions in digestion, absorption, assimilation and elimination. An allergy can also cause impaired functions of the organs and tissues themselves.

In chiropractic theory, an allergy can be seen as a result of a pinched nerve. Impaired functions of the organs and tissues will improve when the pinching of the spinal nerves is removed (by removing the disturbances in the afferent and efferent nerve functions) and energy circulation is restored through chiropractic adjustments. But the adjustments have to be applied on a regular basis. Otherwise the misalignment could return.

I observed this phenomena on my regular chiropractic patients for a long time. I did not have an explanation for the need for "the twice a week" regular chiropractic treatment to keep the body in alignment. Then I combined NAET® with regular chiropractic treatment. When these patients began desensitization for the NAET® basic essential nutrients (NAET® Basic allergens) through NAET®, we noticed that they were holding adjustments for longer times. By the time they completed desensitization on 25 to 30 NAET Basic allergen groups, most of these patients responded very well health-wise. Their chemical sensitivities were reduced greatly and other symptoms also reduced or were eliminated completely. They digested their meals better. Sleep improved. Overall energy increased many fold. Their quality of life improved. They maintained their spinal alignments without losing them so they did not need frequent chiropractic adjustments as before. The observation of these patients invoked enough interest to study the benefits of NAET® on a larger group and we received similar results. From this observation I concluded that allergens are the cause of spinal misalignment, pinched nerves and various other health disorders we see in people.

Oriental medicine explains the same theory from a different perspective. In Oriental medicine, the balance of Yin and Yang represents the perfect balance of energies (the state of homeostasis). Any interference in the energy flow or an energy disturbance can cause an imbalance in the Yin-Yang state and an imbalance in "homeostasis." Any substance that is capable of creating an energy disturbance in one's body is called an allergen.

According to NAET® theory, when a substance is brought into the electromagnetic field of an individual, an attraction or repulsion takes place between the energy of the individual and the substance.

ATTRACTION BETWEEN ENERGIES

If two energies are attracted to each other, both energies benefit each other. The individual can benefit from association with the substance. The energy of the substance will combine with the energy of the individual and enhance functional ability. For example: After taking an antibiotic, the bacterial infection is diminished. Here the energy of the antibiotic joins forces with the energy of the body and helps to eliminate the bacteria. Another example is taking vitamin supplements (if one is not allergic to them) and the gaining of energy and vitality.

REPULSION BETWEEN ENERGIES

If two energies repel each other, they are not good for each other. The individual can experience the repulsion of his/her energy from the other as a discomfort in the body. The energy of the individual will cause energy blockages in his/her energy meridians to prevent invasion of the adverse energy into his/her energy field. For example: After taking a repelling antibiotic, not only does the bacterial infection not get better but the individual might break out in rashes all over the body causing fever, nausea, excessive perspiration, fatigue, etc. If repulsion takes place between two energies, then the substance that is capable of producing the repulsion in a living individual is considered an allergen. When the allergen produces a repulsion of energy in the electromagnetic field, certain energy disturbance takes place in the body. The energy disturbance caused from the repulsion of the substance is capable of producing various unpleasant or adverse reactions. These reactions are considered "allergic reactions."

NATURAL BODY DEFENSE

In certain instances, the body also produces many natural body defenses like "histamine, immunoglobulins, etc." to help the body overcome the unpleasant reactions from interaction with the allergen. The most common immunoglobulin produced during a reaction is called IgE (immunoglobulin E). The activation of IgE antibodies causes what the traditional medical profession calls "true" allergies; however, millions of people experience various allergic symptoms every day in varying degrees without producing these antibodies. These types of reactions can be called either *intolerance* or *hypersensitivity*.

When the body is exposed to what it thinks is a foreign and dangerous substance, a normal immune system will immediately release chemical mediators appropriate to the condition to counteract the allergic reaction. The body will come to a settlement with the allergen in seconds without causing any obvious ill-health symptoms in the body. But when the immune system perceives what should be harmless substances as dangerous intruders and stimulates antibody production to defend the body, things do not settle down as pleasantly as in the individual with a normal immune system. Here, the first contact with an allergen initiates the baby step of an allergic reaction inside the body. The body will alert its defense forces in response to the alarm received about the new invader and will immediately produce a few antibodies, storing them in reserve for future use.

In most cases, a first contact or initial sensitization will usually not produce many symptoms. During the second exposure to the allergen, the body will alert the previously produced antibodies to action, producing more noticeable symptoms. If you have a strong immune system, the second exposure may not cause too many unpleasant symptoms either. But often, with the third exposure, the threatened immune system will begin serious action by producing massive amounts of antibodies to defend against the invader, causing what the traditional allergist calls an allergic reaction.

Various types of immunoglobulins are produced in the body at various times as natural defense mechanisms to protect the body. They include: IgE, IgA, IgD, IgG, and IgM.

Some people could have only the IgE mediated allergies, in which case IgE antibodies can be found in the blood sample. Some others can have more than one antibody in their blood, depending on how many allergens they have reacted to in the past.

People suffer from allergic manifestation in varying degrees because of the above mentioned reasons. Regardless of age, gender, race, or inheritance, anyone can manifest allergies at any time if the circumstances fall within the above causes.

In sensitive individuals, contact with any allergen can produce a variety of symptoms, in varying degrees. The ingested, inhaled or contacted allergens are capable of alerting the body's immune system. The frightened and confused immune system then commands the production and immediate release of immunoglobulins and other chemical mediators.

In order to enjoy life, the chemically sensitive patient must find ways to overcome adverse reactions to the allergens. It can be done easily through NAET®.

NAET® is all about finding the cause and eliminating it permanently so that the symptom arising from that source will disappear forever.

HOME EVALUATION PROCEDURES

Do you suffer from any allergy? Or Allergy-related disorder? Below is an allergy-check list to help you evaluate yourself to see if you have any active or hidden allergies. A sensible solution can be found if you can identify the source of your problem.

Please describe your chief problem in one sentence.

_____

_____

_____

When did your problem begin? Please write approximate date and time if you don't remember the exact date, time and event._____

_____

_____

Rate your symptoms on a scale of 0-10, here "0" equals no symptom or discomfort and "10" equals maximum discomfort.

1. How is your energy at these following hours?

6 am [ ], 8 am [ ], 10 am [ ], 12 noon [ ], 2 PM [ ],
4 PM [ ], 6 PM [ ], 6 PM [ ], 8 PM [ ], 10 PM [ ],
12 am [ ], 2 am [ ], 4 am [ ]

2. How is your appetite? ——————[ ]
3. How is your digestion? —————— [ ]
4. How is your elimination? ——————[ ]
5. How is your sleep? ——————[ ]
6. How is your general well-being? – [ ]

ORGAN-MERIDIAN ASSOCIATION TIME

It takes two hours to circulate energy through one energy meridian. If the energy can travel through the meridians without any obstruction in the flow, you should feel good overall. If there is any energy disturbance in the meridian, it will reflect on your health depending on the meridian(s) affected. If you feel unusual symptoms or illnesses, note the time of the day you felt differently. After you find the time, find the corresponding meridian (s) from the list below.

NAMES OF THE MERIDIANS

Lung (Lu) .... 3-5 am

Large Intestine (LI) .... 5-7 am

Stomach (St) .... 7-9 am

Spleen (Sp) 9-11am

Heart (Ht) ....11-1 pm

Small Intestine - (SI).......1-3 pm

Urinary Bladder (UB)......3-5 pm

Kidney (Ki) ....5-7 pm

Pericardium (PC or CI)...7-9 pm

Triple warmer (TW)........9-11pm

Gall Bladder (GB)..........11-1 am

Liver (Lv).......................1-3 am

Then go to Chapter 4 in this book to find out more about your health. Detailed information about the normal and abnormal functions of the acupuncture meridians is given in Chapter 4. If there is no energy blockage in the meridian(s), then an individual will experience normal functions. In the case of an energy blockage(s), abnormal function(s) can be seen or experienced by the individual. Then go to Chapter 6 to learn the home-balancing techniques. Do it once or twice a day for a few weeks. No matter what condition you are in, your home-balancing treatment will make a difference in your overall health. If the problem is mild you should be able to help eliminate your problem by simply following

ORGAN CLOCK INDICATING TIMES OF GREATEST ACTIVITY

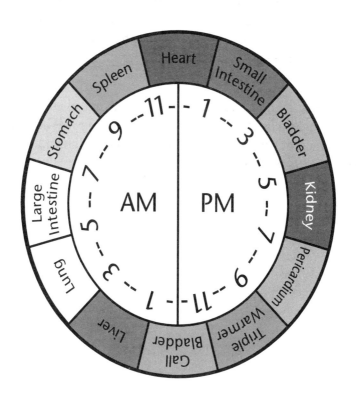

YIN/YANG

the home-balancing procedures given in Chapter 6. But if the problem is more than mild, please find a NAET® specialist immediately and have the doctor evaluate your condition and do further necessary treatments. We have received numerous testimonials from many users of home-help procedures that by massaging these balancing points on a regular basis, they have been able to maintain better health.

Please read through the next few pages and evaluate yourself to make a list of possible sensitivities. You will be able to detect most of your sensitivities by yourself if you go through this self-evaluation of your symptoms.

ALLERGY SYMPTOM CHECKLIST

Please read the following list of symptoms in the next few pages. They could be caused from allergies. Many thousands of people have received relief from these symptoms by treating with NAET®. Please rate your symptoms on a scale of 0-3: (0= no symptoms; 1= mild symptoms; 2= moderate symptoms; 3= severe symptoms).

RATING   SYMPTOMS

— Acne

— Addiction to alcohol

— Addiction to caffeine

— Addiction to chocolate

— Addiction to coffee

— Addiction to drugs

— Addiction to food

— Addiction to smoking

— Addiction to sugar

— Addictions to carbohydrate

— Aggression

— Allergy to animals

— Allergy to aspirin

— Allergy to insects

— Allergy to cold

— Allergy to corn

— Allergy to Fish

— Allergy to shellfish

RATING   SYMPTOMS

— Allergy to food additives

— Allergy to food colorings

— Allergy to gasoline

— Allergy to hair dye

— Allergy to heat

— Allergy to humidity

— Allergy to latex

— Allergy to mercury

— Allergy to milk products

— Allergy to mushroom

— Allergy to mold

— Allergy to newspaper ink

— Allergy to nuts

— Allergy to paper

— Allergy to penicillin

— Allergy to perfume

— Allergy to plastics

— Allergy to pollens

— Allergy to proteins

— Allergy to radiation

— Allergy to razor blade

— Allergy to salt

— Allergy to smells

— Allergy to sugar

— Allergy to trees

RATING   SYMPTOMS

- Allergy to weeds
- Allergy to wheat/gluten
- Amnesia temporary
- Anemia
- Angina-like pains
- Anxiety attacks
- Arthritis
- Asthma, bronchial
- Asthma, cardiac
- Athletes foot
- Attention deficit disorder
- Backache
- Bone pains
- Bipolar disorders
- Biting nails
- Blurred vision
- Bowel disorder
- Brain fog
- Breast-pain
- Burning feet
- Burning in the groin
- Burning sensation on urination
- Candida/yeast
- Canker sores
- Cardiac arrhythmia

RATING   SYMPTOMS

— Cervical dysplasia

— Chronic cough

— Chronic low grade fever

— Chronic nasal congestion

— Clumsiness

— Cold extremities

— Cold intolerance

— Cold sores

— Colitis

— Compulsive behavior

— Constipation

— Craving fat

— Craving spices

— Craving salt

— Craving sour

— Craving sweets

— Craving bitters

— Craving onions

— Crohns' disease

— Conjunctivitis

— Cuts heal slowly

— Dandruff

— Decreased sex drive

— Dermatitis

— Depression

RATING   SYMPTOMS

— Diabetes

— Diarrhea

— Difficulty in walking

— Difficulty in swallowing

— Distractibility

— Diverticulitis

— Dizziness

— Dream disturbed sleep

— Dry eyes

— Dry mouth

— Dry skin

— Dryness

— Dyslexia

— Earaches

— Ear infections

— Eating dirt

— Eating disorders

— Eczema

— Edema of the feet

— Elbow pain

— Eyelids puffy

— Emphysema

— Enuresis (bed wetting)

— Erratic disruptive behavior

— Excessive appetite

RATING   SYMPTOMS

— Excessive drooling

— Excessive flatulence

— Excessive salivation

— Excessive sweating

— Exercise-induced asthma

— Failing memory

— Fainting spells

— Fatigue

— Fever of unknown origin

— Feels insecure

— Fibromyalgia

— Fibrocystic breast

— Food craving

— Food sensitivity

— Forgetfulness

— Formaldehyde allergy

— Frequent repetitive activity

— Frequent bronchitis

— Frequent ear infection

— Frequent flu's and colds.

— Frequent infections

— Frequent pneumonia

— Frequent sore throat

— Frequent sweating

— Frequent urination

RATING   SYMPTOMS

— Gags easily

— Gallstones

— Gastric distress

— Gastric ulcer

— General body aches

— General fatigue

— General itching

— Glaucoma

— Greasy food upsets

— Groin pain

— Growing pains

— Hay-fever

— Hair loss

— Hair pulling

— Halitosis

— Hand flicking

— Head banging

— Headache/afternoon

— Headache/migraine

— Headache over the eyes

— Headaches/sinus

— Headache/morning

— Headaches under the eyes

— Hearing loss

— Hearing decreased

RATING   SYMPTOMS

— Heartburn

— Heart irregularities

— Hemorrhoids

— Herpes Genital

— Herpes Zoster

— Hepatitis

— High altitude problem

— High blood pressure

— High cholesterol

— Hives

— Hoarseness

— Holds on to people and objects.

— Hot flashes

— Hungry between meals

— Hyperactivity

— Hypoglycemia

— Impaired ability to role-play

— Impaired speech

— Impaired peer relationships

— Impulsivity

— Increased sex drive

— Increased thirst

— Indigestion

— Infertility

— Internal tremor

RATING   SYMPTOMS

— Insomnia

— Irregular periods

— Irritability

— Irritable bowels

— Itchy eyes

— Jock itch

— Joint pains

— Keyed up, fails to calm

— Knee pains

— Labored breathing

— Leaky gut syndrome

— Learning disabilities

— Light sensitivity

— Listlessness

— Loss of taste
— Loose stools

— Loud talk

— Low backache

— Low blood pressure

— Low body temperature

— Low libido

— Lump in the breast

— Lump in the throat

— Lupus

— Lymph node tenderness

— Metallic taste in the mouth

RATING   SYMPTOMS

- — Mid backache
- — Migrating pains
- — Milk causes discomfort
- — Mood swings
- — Mucus in the throat
- — Multiple sclerosis
- — Muscle cramps at night
- — Muscle pain
- — Muscle spasms
- — Nasal polyps
- — Nausea
- — Neck pains
- — Nervous stomach
- — Neuralgia
- — Night sweats
- — Nosebleed
- — Neuropathies
- — Numbness anywhere in the body
- — Obsessive behavior
- — Ovarian cyst
- — Pain between shoulders
- — Pain on the heels
- — Pain anywhere in the body without reason
- — Panic attacks
- — Paranoia

RATING   SYMPTOMS

- — Parasitic infestation
- — Parrot-like talking
- — Phobias
- — Picking at skin.
- — Pre menstrual pains or discomfort
- — Poor appetite
- — Poor concentration
- — Poor memory
- — Post nasal drip
- — Premature graying
- — Prone to infections
- — Prostate troubles
- — Psoriasis
- — Recurrent prostatitis
- — Red blood cells low
- — Red blood cells high
- — Red eyes
- — Repeated dental infection
- — Restless leg syndrome
- — Reflex sympathetic dystrophy
- — Ring worm
- — Ringing in the ears
- — Sadness
- — Sand-like feeling in the eyes
- — Sciatic neuralgia

RATING   __SYMPTOMS__

— Scleroderma

— Seizures

— Sensitivities to any chemicals

— Sensitive to cold

— Sensitive to heat

— Sensitivities to weather change

— Shoulder pain

— Short term memory loss

— Shortness of breath

— Sighs frequently

— Sinusitis

— Skin problems

— Sleep apnea

— Sleepy during the day

— Slow pulse

— Slow starter

— Smell-decreased

— Sneezing attacks

— Sore throat

— Startles easily

— Strokes

— Strong lights irritates

— Swollen joints, ankles

— Thickening skin

— Thinning skin

RATING   SYMPTOMS

— Throat constriction

— Thyroid problem

— Tightness in the chest

— Tingling around the mouth

— Tingling anywhere in the body

— Tourette's syndrome

— Tires too easily

— Toxicity to heavy metal

— Toxicity to pesticides

— Ulcerative colitis

— Uncontrollable body movements

— Unable to fall asleep at night

— Unable to go back to sleep upon wakening

— Unable to sleep for long hours without waking

— Unexplained chest pain

— Unexplained pain in the body

— Unreasonable anger

— Unrefreshing sleep

— Unusual weight loss

— Upper backaches

— Urinary tract disorder

— Urination difficult

— Urine amount decreased

— Urine amount increased

— Uterine polyp

RATING   SYMPTOMS

— Vaginal discharge

— Varicose veins

— Vision problems

— Vomiting frequently

— Vulvodynia

— Vertigo

— Warts

— Weak nails

— Wake up during the night

— Watery eyes

— Weight gain for no reason

— Weight loss

— White blood cells low

— White blood cells high

— White spots

— Worrier

— Yeast infections

— Other

2

A chemically sensitive individual can react to multi tudes of items from his/her surroundings. We have reached the age of modern living through chemistry or , as the TV ads said in the late 1940's and early 1950's, "Better living through Chemistry." What has happened in modern industrial society, however, is the misuse, overuse, and inappropriate disposal of chemicals. We now know from our experience that many of these chemicals can be toxic. Some harmful exposures are from ignorance, some from oversight, and some are from criminal negligence (Our toxic world - by Doris Rapp, 2003). The result on individuals, certain groups who suffer from never ending allergic reactions is toxic injury. Toxic exposure, whether acute or chronic, creates an overload of the toxins on the individual which can result in serious health problems (Chernoff, A Daily Dose of Toxin, 2005).

What is Chemical Sensitivity?
A condition of unusual sensitivity of an individual to one or more chemicals (man-made chemical or seen naturally occurring in the environment) to which the majority of other individuals may

be nonsensitive or nonreactive. The National Research Council, 1992 workshop on Multiple Chemical Sensitivities (a group working on research protocols for clinical evaluation) reported in Toxicology and Industrial Health [Vol. 10 number 4/5 July - October, 1994 Pg. 259 in Claudia Miller's article] the definition of MCS by the National Research Counsel, 1992: Chemical Sensitivity: By sensitivity we mean symptoms or signs as related to chemical exposures at levels tolerated by the population at large, that is distinct from such well recognized hypersensitivity phenomenon as IgG-mediated immediate hypersensitivity reactions, contact dermatitis, and hypersensitivity triggered pneumonitis. Sensitivity may be expressed as symptoms and signs in one or more organ systems.

What is Multiple Chemical Sensitivity (MCS)?

A condition of unusual sensitivity of an individual to more than one chemicals (man-made chemical or seen naturally occurring in the environment) to which the majority of other individuals may be nonsensitive or nonreactive. Cullin, M.R. ed. (1987) "Workers with multiple chemical sensitivities" Occupational Medicine; State of the Art Reviews, defines multiple chemical sensitivity (MCS) as an acquired disorder characterized by recurrent symptoms referable to multiple organ systems, occurring in response to demonstrable exposure to many chemically unrelated compounds at doses far below those established in the general population to cause harmful effects. No single widely accepted test of physiological function can be shown to correlate with these symptoms. [Cullen, M.R. (1987). The Worker with multiple chemical sensitivities: an overview. In Cullen, M.R. (ed). Occupational Medicine: State of the Art Reviews. Hanley and Belfus, Philadelphia. 655-662]

Exposure to any of these items can produce debilitating symptoms in chemically sensitive people. Some of these symptoms are also listed in the pages 54-55. Very often these symptoms are diagnosed at their face value and the original cause of chemical sensitivity is overlooked.

Commonly Seen Triggers of Sensitivity Reaction in Chemically Sensitive People

Acrylic nails
After-shave lotion
Anything around the bed
Alarm clock
Alcoholic beverages
Air pollution
Air filters
Air purifiers
Amalgam
Antiperspirants
Aroma
Asbestos
Aspartame
Aluminum
Antibiotics
Anti-depressants
Air conditioners
Anti-bacterials
Alcohol
Automobile exhaust
Auto-detailing chemicals
Bacteria
Batteries

Bath accessories
Bedroom materials
Bed
Bed frame
 Bed linen
Bed pillow
Bed pillow cover
Benzene
Bleach
Benzyl benzoate
Body wash
Body creme
Body and hand lotion
Brominated compounds
Boron
Borax
Bodycare products
Books
Building materials
Chemicals from work or home
(kitchen, bathroom, and pool),
cosmetics
Cars

Chlorine
Chloramines
Cleanliness
Charcoal
Candida
Carpets
Carpet chemicals
Car smell
Carbon monoxide
Carbon dioxide
Carcinogens
Clorox
Chlorine dioxide
Caffeine
Camphor
Central heating
Car deodorizer
Ceramic tiles
Cooking smells
Crude oil
Dandruff
Dander
Deodorants
Dioxins
Drinks
Drinking water
Detergents
Down pillow
Dry wall material
Dry cleaning chemicals
Dust mites
Dishwashing liquid

Water dechlorinating salts
Dyes
DDT
Diesel
Deodorizers
Dish washing soap
Dust and dustmites
House dust
Industrial dust
Carpet dust
Flour dust (used in baking and cooking)
Talcum powder
Electromagnetic radiation
Environmental substances (grass, weeds, trees, pollens, flowers, sand)
Fabrics
Fabric softeners
Face cream
Fluoride
Flame retardents
Flavored drinks
Fresh food
Food combining
Foods from other source (TV dinners, instant soups)
Monosodium glutamate [msg]
aspartame
Food colorings
Food additives
Food flavorings

Food chemicals
Shelf-life enhancers
Taste enhancers
Appearance enhancers
Foods with chemical sprays
Formaldehyde
Food coloring
Fibreglass
Fumes
Fumigants
Fungi
Fragrances
Gasoline
Geopathic stress
Genetically modified
Glossy paper
Gloss-finished brochures
Glossy pictures and photos
Glues
Hair spray
Headboard
Heavy metals
Herbs and spices
Herbicides
Handwashing soap
Housecleaning chemicals
House-plants
Insulation
Indoor pollution
Industrial waste
Insect bites and stings
Insecticides

In-car pollution
Immunization
Irritants
Cleansing supplies
Jams
Jelly and marmalades
Jewelry
Kava kava
Kelp
Lead
Laminates
Latex (elastics, stretch pants, socks, cosmetic applicators, gloves
Fillers in seats and cushions of sofa and cars, stuffed toys and pillow fillers, linoleum) laundry room
Low level ozone
Lints
Medications (prescription medication, over-the-counter medication, medicinal skin creams)
Mobile phones
Mobile phone accessories
Mercury
Microwaves
Magnets
Mattresses
Milk and milk products
Moth repellants

Freedom From Chemical Sensitivities

Mothballs
Mold
Mold spores
Moss
Methylene chloride
Methanol
Mannitol
Microorganisms (bacteria, viruses, parasites)
Mouthwash
Nickel
Naphthalene
New car smell
Noxious fumes
Noxious chemicals
Natural products
Natural handwash
Natural dishwashing liquid
Nicotine
Nuclear power
Natural cosmetics
Natural paints
Natural toothpowder
Organophosphates
Organic food
Organic clothing
Organic products
Organic paints
Ozone
Oils
Office products
Office machines
Office furniture
Paint
Paint thinner
Pajamas
Packaging material
Plastic toys
Polyvinyl chloride
PCB's (polychlorinated biphenyl) pbb (polybrominated bipnenyl)
pesticides
Pets
Phenylalanine
Paper products (newspaper, toilet paper, books, bills, paper money)
Paint
Paraffins
Perfumes
Plastics (household products, house-wares, utility products, cosmetic applicators, phones, computer, key board, mouse, mouse pad, containers, electrical outlet covers, lids of vitamin containers, hard plastics, soft plastics, saran wrap, freezer bags, shopping bags, and various types of bags)
Picture frame on the wall
Phosphates

Pollen
Pollutants
Potpourri
Polystyrene
Paint strippers
Photocopiers
Preservatives
Pressed wood
Quartz
Quartz crystals
Radon
Refrigerators
Recycled paper goods
Recycling
Radiation
Radioactivity
Radiators
Soap
Solvents
Sweeteners
Saccharin
Salt
Sugar
Saturated fats
Shampoo
Smog
Soft drinks
Sweat-rash
Static
Static ions
Static electricity
Scents

Scrubbers (foam, metal, vinyl or plastic scrubbers in the kitchen)
Shampoo and hair conditioners
Sorbitol
Sulphates
Stabilisers
Synthetic detergents
Synthetic materials (polyester, acrylic, acetate, nylon, cotton, rayon, silk, other petrochemical-based fabrics, rugs and carpet)
Silica
Silicates
Smells from various sources (from cooking, frying, seasoning, perfume, outside air, bodily secretion, or discharge, body odor, decayed material, stale food, flowers, perfume or any smell of cosmetics from the bed partner, hospital wards, changed dressings from surgical wounds, (water from gutters), (backwaters), smell of waste products, smell of stool, other discharge)
Supplements (vitamins, minerals, diet products, herbal and homeopathic remedies

and other supplements)
Tap water
Toothpaste
Turpentine
Tertrazine
Tetevision sets
Television remote control
Toxic fumes
Toxic chemicals
Trihalomethane
Ultra-violet radiation
Uranium

Utensils
Varnish
Vaccines
Vinyl
Volatile organic compounds
Wood works and products
Wood furniture
Cane products
Wood cabinet
Wood tables
wooden cutting board
Wooden floor

A major health problems seen in chemically sensitive people is:

Upper Respiratory Disorders

Asthma
Emphysema
Bronchitis
Chronic lung disorders
Hay-fever
Rhinitis

Sinusitis
Sinus infection
Chronic cough
Post nasal drip
Throat rritation
Seasonal allergies

OTHER DISORDERS

Acne
ADD & ADHD
Addictions
Allergic dermatitis
Anxiety
Arthritis
Atopic dermatitis
Autism
Cancer
Candida infections (Candidiasis)
Cardiovascular disorders
Chemical sensitivities
Chronic fatigue syndrome
Chronic infections
Circulatory disorders
Depression
Digestive disorders
Ear troubles
Eczema
Emotional imbalances
Emphysema
Endocrine disorders
Eye disorders
Fibromyalgia
Food allergy
Food intolerances
General body ache
Genitourinary disorders
Geopathic stress
Gulf-war syndrome
Headache
Hormonal imbalances
Hyperactivity
Immune system disorders
Inflammatory conditions
Insomnia
Infertility
Irritable bowel syndrome
Itchy scalp
Itchy skin
Joint disorders
Loss of hair
Mental disorders
Nutritional disorders
Parasitic infestations
Post viral syndrome
Psoriasis
Reactions to vaccines and
Immunizations
Seasonal affective disorders
Seasonal allergies
Sick building syndrome
Skin disorders
Sleep disorders
Tumors
Various emotional imbalances
Yeast infection
Other types of pain disorders

Categories of Allergies

Allergic reactions can be grouped according to the clinical manifestations of the person with allergies.

1. People suffering from food allergies:

They have no seasonal symptoms, but suffer from varying numbers of unusual or unpleasant physical, physiological or emotional symptoms whenever they eat any food with some chemicals (for example, foods prepared with colorings, food additives, monosodium glutamate, etc.).

2. People suffering from chemical allergies through external sources:

They have no unusual symptoms if they do not come in contact with any chemicals. They can be happy and healthy when they live in a natural environment surrounded by natural life, eating organically grown, unprocessed food. But, whenever they come near or in contact with any chemicals they are sensitive to, they suffer from a varying number of unusual or unpleasant physical, physiological, or emotional symptoms. As long as they wear or use 100% cotton, silk or any natural fabrics, they function well.

3. People suffering from chemical allergies from internal sources:

This group of people react to their own body secretions (sweat, urine, feces, mucous, semen, tears and saliva), body parts (hair and nails), different organs (stomach, spleen, lungs, kidney, liver, heart, brain, etc.). The body's defense mechanism is derailed, and the body makes antibodies against its own tissues and/or fluids. The immune system attacks the body that it inhabits, which eventually causes damage or alteration to its own cells, tissues, organs and functions. Such damage results in cancer, abnormal tissue growths and tumors, kidney failure, organ failure, hearing loss, poor vision, heart attacks, liver failure, cataract, adrenal depletion, diabetes, thyroid malfunctions, etc.

4.   People allergic to natural environmental allergens:

These people have frequent tearing from the eyes, sneezing, wheezing, have asthma and other upper respiratory disturbances, suffer from fatigue, irritability and hay-fever symptoms during pollen season (pollens from weeds, trees, flowers and grasses), allergic to cotton, natural materials, but feel reasonably well for the rest of the year if they avoid natural products made from natural substances.

5.   People suffering from allergies to animals and other humans:

These people have no allergies to food, drinks or the materials around them. They react to the electromagnetic energy of other living beings, which makes them allergic to other human beings, like their mother, father, spouse, brother, sister, children, partners, employee and employer. They can also have allergies to pets, cats, dogs, insects, bees, ants, etc.

6   People with emotional allergies:

The people in this group have allergies to the actions and interactions of everyday life. They may be allergic to their own: thoughts or feelings (fear, anger, self-esteem, creativity, power, self-worth, inferiority, superiority, etc.); concepts: ("I can never get healthy," "I can never lose weight," or "I can never make enough money," etc.); a memory of a certain incidence (such as nightmares, fear or anxiety while driving due to a memory of a highway auto accident that happened 10 years ago); emotions, like hating jobs or obsessions with careers (teaching, acting, cooking, gardening, writing, shopping, shop-lifting, etc.), and interactions (fighting with co-workers, classmates, boss or teachers). Some allergic people enjoy going against rules and regulations, acting against the norm in situations or disobeying authorities (running red lights when the police is not watching, etc.)

7.   People with combination allergies:

This group of people react to what seems to be an infinite number of combinations of food, pollens, chemicals, other humans, animals, thoughts, memories and concepts.

8.   People who are universal reactors:

This group has multiple chemical sensitivities and suffers from severe reactions to all of the above allergens. They generally suffer from many other health problems. They are grouped as ecologically and environmentally ill. Ecological illness is the result of adverse reactions to substances in the air, water, food, living environment, work environments, and chemicals. These people do not feel safe anywhere. They can suffer from varied, chronic symptoms listed in page 54. These are the people who some-times need to live in a protective "bubble."

It is rare to see people fall in any one group. Usually, people suffer symptoms from two or more groups.

CATEGORIES OF ALLERGENS

Common allergens are generally classified into nine basic categories based primarily on the method in which they are con-tacted, rather than the symptoms they produce.

1. Inhalants

2. Ingestants

3. Contactants

4. Injectants

5. Infectants

6. Physical agents

7. Genetic factors

8. Molds and fungi

9. Emotional Stressors

INHALANTS

Inhalants are those allergens that are contacted through the nose, throat and bronchial tubes. Examples of inhalants are mi-croscopic spores of certain grasses, flowers, pollens, powders, smoke, cosmetics, perfumes; and chemical fumes such as paint, insecticides, fertilizers, flour from grains, cooking smells, etc.

It is difficult to say that there is a typical or predictable allergic reaction, or set of reactions, in response to a given allergen. If there is a predictable response, however, it is in this general category of inhalants that it comes closest to being found.

Most of us have suffered the discomfort that comes from accidentally breathing a toxic substance. For example, when we smell chlorine gas from a bottle of common household bleach, our reaction is immediate and violent as our eyes water, noses run, and bronchial tubes go into spasm, making breathing difficult. This experiment can be duplicated over and over if we want a proof that bleach is directly responsible for a given set of reactions. Of course, most of us learn very quickly that it is the bleach that caused our discomfort, and we decide to be more careful in the future.

In this case, the cause of the discomfort (the bleach) was very closely associated with the effect the burning eyes, runny nose, and restricted breathing. A simple and very scientific deduction, though slightly sophomoric in this context, can be drawn from this cause-and-effect relationship. A proper diagnosis based on a similar cause-and-effect relationship is much more difficult when the cause is olive pollen, encountered early in the day by one of the sensitive patients, and the resultant delayed effect is similar to that experienced when one breathes in the bleach. Similarly, hay fever is generally the result of breathing the spores of pollinating grass and weeds. It normally occurs when these plants are in bloom in the spring or, in warmer climates, closely following a summer rain and the resultant regrowth of the grasses and weeds on the hillsides. Sinus drainage and restricted breathing are the direct and reproducible results of an allergic reaction to an inhalant.

Consider how much more difficult it is to make a proper diagnosis when the patient's physical responses to a given allergen differ radically from those that would normally be anticipated.

A three-year-old girl suffered from early morning asthma. She woke up about 6:00 am and began coughing and wheezing. Quite often her parents had to rush her to the emergency room when she does not respond to the nebulizer or sprays. Her mysterious asthma worried the doctor and her parents. Then she was referred to me by her doctor. In the office when I evaluated her with NST, the cause was traced to something she was smelling. She had many allergies including milk, nuts, fish, etc. So we continued to treat her for the basics. After her basics her mother expressed her desire to treat her for chocolate since she was fond of chocolate and they were not giving her due to her allergies. After the chocolate treatment the whole family was instructed not to use coffee or chocolate in any form. Every morning her father brewed coffee around 6:00 a.m. before he went to work. The aroma of the coffee woke up the girl and produced asthma because she was highly allergic to the smell of the coffee. So the day after the treatment little Faye didn't have any cough or asthma. But the following day she woke up again with coughing and asthma. She was only treated for the energy of the coffee and chocolate. The girl was in fact allergic to the smell. So I had to ask the mother to bring in brewed coffee for her to get treated for the smell. Mission was successful. After that treatment, she did not have morning asthma anymore.

This clearly points out that there is no typical response to allergens in the real world. If we are depending on allergies to produce a given set of responses for all people, we may misdiagnose and provide wrong treatments. We must remember that since we cannot duplicate and package a cause-and-effect responsive medication as antidote to handle all cases of poisoning from inhaling fern tree spores, or any other allergen, we must not over-simplify our treatment of patients who do not exhibit typical allergic symptoms, whatever we perceive them to be. Otherwise, we risk missing myriad potential reactions that may be produced in some people in response to their contacts with substances that are, for them, allergens.

HAY-FEVER AND ALLERGIC RHINITIS

Hay Fever describes the symptoms of allergic rhinitis when it occurs in the late summer due to an individual's reaction to ragweeds and sage weeds or fresh flowers and grasses. Allergic rhinitis affects an estimated 40-50 million people in the United States. It is a very common medical problem affecting more than 15 percent of the population, both adults and children. Allergic rhinitis takes two different forms, seasonal and perennial. Symptoms of seasonal allergic rhinitis occur in spring, summer and/or early fall and are usually caused by allergic sensitivity to pollens from trees, grasses, weeds or to airborne mold spores. Other people experience symptoms year-round, a condition called perennial allergic rhinitis. It is generally caused by sensitivity to house dust, dust mites, animal dander and mold spores. Food allergies are another possible cause. Most hay fever sufferers feel better in warm, sunny weather. This condition frequently causes the patient to feel chills almost constantly. As a result, hay fever patients require more bedding and warmer clothing when suffering from this ailment. Hay fever and allergic rhinitis are both characterized by symptoms of watery discharge from the nose, eyes, and throat, loss of taste and smell, and other symptoms similar to those accompanying colds. The three most common symptoms are severe sneezing, watery nasal discharge, and stuffy nose. Many patients also complain of an annoying tickle inside the nose that results in violent sneezing. Others have dry, hacking coughs, and some have a profuse watery secretion of the nasal passages.

Many patients with pollen allergies will also be allergic to certain foods, as well as to other inhalants and contactants. Other than pollens and grasses, the most common items found to cause hay fever are: sugar, carob, corn, wheat, beans, pineapple, tomato, banana, perfume, furniture, cats, dogs, feathers, kapok, dust, plastics, rubber and leather. Often, hay fever victims also suffer from nasal polyps, which are swellings or growths of the mucus membrane that occur within the nostrils. Nasal polyps are caused by congestion and inflammation of the mucous membrane and tend to grow or shrink in accordance with the severity of the symptoms. In some instances, they become large enough to completely block the nasal passages and even extend beyond the nostrils.

It is extremely important that hay fever sufferers consult an appropriate allergist knowledgeable in NAET when their symptoms begin. Hay fever has a tendency to become increasingly severe with each season. The possibility of serious complications increases with each severe hay fever attack. Untreated patients are also likely to accumulate new allergens, as well as encountering increased sensitivity in their reactions.

Allergic rhinitis may be caused by other substances including house dust, occupational dusts (such as flour in the bakery, industrial dust), chalk powder, newspaper ink, paint, plastics, chemical sprays, soaps, perfumes and other chemical agents.

Prompt treatment of these allergies greatly decreases the likelihood that a comparatively mild allergic manifestation, such as hay-fever or allergic rhinitis, will develop into a more severe allergy, such as asthma.

ASTHMA

Asthma is the 9th leading cause of hospitalization nationally. Over one billion dollars is spent each year on health care for asthma in the U.S.

An allergic tendency toward asthma (although not the actual allergic disease) is inherited. It occurs much more frequently in families that have a history of various allergic conditions. The tendency toward this particular allergic ailment seems to be more frequently inherited than in most other allergic diseases. A woman who suffers from hay fever may have children who suffer from some other manifestations, such as dermatitis (rather than hay fever). On the other hand, a patient who suffers from asthma is quite likely to have children who also suffer from asthma.

Allergens, like pollens, flowers, molds and dusts are the most prevalent cause of asthmatic attacks. In addition, asthma can be caused by allergies to almost any: food (fish, shellfish, peanuts, food additives, food colors, sulfites), clothing, chemicals (fabric softeners, detergents, shampoo, body lotion), perfumes, synthetic substances (plastics, latex, rubber goods, ceramics, tiles, cookware) and natural substances (cotton, leather). Cold, heat, dampness and moisture can cause an asthmatic reaction as well as an allergy to one's spouse, children or another human associate, even, a pet.

Like other allergic conditions, asthma responds very well to NAET. When beginning treatment, it is always better to combine Western medical treatments with NAET for better and faster results. After you are treated for the basic items, you can evaluate your symptoms and try to gradually reduce the dosage of any medication that you may be taking.

Asthmatics should always carry inhalant sprays for quick relief in emergencies because an asthmatic attack can be triggered at any time from an unexpected contact with an allergen (please read Say Good-bye to Asthma by the author if you would like to learn more about NAET asthma care).

Many people are allergic to the medication they take for relief. When they do not receive the expected relief from their medication, they complain to their doctors. Doctors will change to a different medication and if that doesn't work, move on to another. The doctor's and the patient's frustration can be reduced by learning NAET testing techniques or neuromuscular sensitivity testing (NST). Doctors could check the medication through NST before prescribing it. Pharmacists could check the allergy before they supply the medication to the patient. It is very essential to teach NST to all practicing medical professionals and pharmacists. You (the patient or guardian) should also learn the testing techniques in order to test yourself for the medications you are taking. You can screen allergy to the medication before you take them. This way, you can eliminate the frustration of seeking different doctors and different remedies.

SINUSITIS

Sinusitis is inflammation or infection of any of the four groups of sinus cavities in the skull, which open into the nasal passages. Sinusitis is not the same as rhinitis, although the two may be associated and their symptoms may be similar. The terms "sinus trouble" or "sinus congestion" are sometimes wrongly used to mean congestion of the nasal passages. Most cases of nasal congestion are not associated with sinusitis. If sinusitis is allowed to continue, it can eventually turn into asthma.

COUGH VARIANT ASTHMA

Cough variant asthma is seen among children. Cough is the main noticeable symptom among little children. They may be normal during the day. But when they go to bed they begin coughing. Eventually their coughing will end up in wheezing and shortness of breath.

In these children, a major culprit may be traced to something in the bed. Bedroom materials can cause cough asthma not only in children, even in adults too. The common allergens causing cough and asthma at night, especially in bed: bed linen, detergent, mattress, pesticides and chemicals seen in the mattress, pillow, pillow case, stuffed toys, plastic toys, plastic sheets, crib toys, reading books, remote control for the TV, pajama, other night wear clothes, socks, tooth brush, tooth paste, mouth wash, tap water, the night air, night blooming plants if the window is left open, house plants in the bed room, bed room furniture, curtains, drapes, carpets, ceramic tiles, bathroom slippers, depending on what kind of materials one has in the bedroom.

A 5-year-old young boy suffered from severe cough through the night. When I evaluated him in my office NST detected that he was reacting to the paintings parents had stored under his bed in cardboard boxes. He was allergic to the dried up paint thinner in the paintings. Even though it was an old painting, energy of the paint thinner was still on the painting and for a sensitive person, the dried up paint was enough to trigger an allergic reaction.

People love eating chocolates and enjoy drinking coffee and other caffeinated drinks. Many people are allergic to chocolate and coffee and in them allergy to these items produce asthma.

Sam, age 42, had a throat irritation and cough that always started at 4 p.m. and subsided by 8 p.m. He worked as a travel agent, and his busy hours were 4-6 p.m. His irritating cough made him very uncomfortable. After proper evaluation, it was discovered that he ate a certain brand of chocolate candy bar every day at 2 p.m. during his break. By 4 p.m., the allergic reaction from the candy bar showed up as coughing spells. After treatment for chocolate, he never had the problem again.

A nurse, 43 came in with a strange problem. During the day she suffered from cough and asthma. In spite of her asthma medication, she continued to cough and wheeze through the day. She worked day shift, which started from 7:00 am and ended at 7:00 p.m. As soon as she reached home, she removed her worked clothes and settled in comfortable home clothes. She attributed her cough and asthma to the various smells in the hospital where she worked. I treated her for the NAET basics, she felt better overall. But asthma did not reduce. After the basics, she was evaluated again and detected that she was reacting to her synthetic bra. On questioning her she told me that she never wore a bra at home. She put it on only when she went to work or to visit friends or family. After she was treated for her bra, she stopped having asthma.

COOKING PANS INDUCED DISORDERS

Cooking pans, Teflon coating on the pans, cooking sprays, kitchen materials like scrubbers, dishwashing soap, smells from: cooking, frying and seasoning, burnt food, popcorn popping, coffee brewing, meat cooking, old kitchen trash, spoiled food, rancid oils, unclean garbage disposal, cleaning chemicals, etc., can produce respiratory symptoms (asthma, sinusitis, coughing spells, dusty feeling in the throat, hay fever-like symptoms and sensation of choking) in sensitive individuals.

For her whole life, a 54-year-old housewife who loved to cook could not tolerate the smell of fried oil. Whenever she smelled any deep-fried food, she ended up with severe asthma. She was treated in our office for heated oils. Now, not only can she smell the oil, but she can also cook and eat with the family without having any trace of upper respiratory problems.

A 27-year-old newly married man suffered from severe asthma whenever he had intercourse with his wife. He was allergic to her vaginal secretion and the smell of it. After the problem was identified and treated, he did not suffer from asthma anymore.

A newly married woman suffered from throat infection, cough that eventually turned into asthma, and weeping ulcers through out her body. NAET testing detected that her body is allergic to saliva. She did not have any cats or dogs or other pets since she had known to be allergic to them. On questioning her regarding any possibility of exposure to some saliva, she blushed and kept silent. I didn't know how to treat her not knowing the source. Finally, she said her husband licked her entire body before they made love every time. She was simply allergic to his saliva as well as semen. She was treated several times for his saliva and semen before she completely became symptom-free.

We had several women allergic to their husband's semen, urine and saliva. Some suffered from severe yeast-like infection that did not respond to any medication. When they were treated for the semen, their yeast-infection said good-bye to them.

I have treated many men and women who developed multiple chemical sensitivities after they got married. The culprits were traced to the partner's clothes, perfume, hair sprays, after-shave, body odor, etc.

CIGARETTE SMELL

The smell of cigarette smoke can trigger sensitivity reactions in chemically sensitive individuals. Such people have to isolate in their own house most of the time. They cannot go out in crowds, to movies, or in shopping malls, airplanes, entertainment parks, restaurants, etc., for fear of asthmatic attacks. Lately, smoking is restricted in many areas in this country. Even so, smokers find their ways to pollute public areas with smoke, making it hard for smoke-sensitive individuals to live a normal life. NAET can eliminate the allergy to smoke so asthmatics can survive in smoky neighborhoods.

If you are sensitive to smoke, you might also be sensitive to other fumes in the air. Fireplace smoke, smell from coffee brewing, popcorn popping, cooking smell, smell from gasoline, automobile exhaust, etc., can also be trigger for chemical sensitivity reaction.

It is helpful to use air purifiers in the house if you are sensitive to these smells. There are many chemical and odor free products available to help alleviate your symptoms. During the initial NAET treatments, such aids will be beneficial.

Emotional factors can also trigger cough, asthma, sinusitis, bronchitis, upper respiratory disorders, pain disorders and insomnia, etc. Emotional upsets, such as death, divorce, problem at work, or in the family, even unresolved arguments can produce respiratory problems like cough, sinusitis, asthma, shortness of breath, blocked nostrils, etc. and various other physical or physiologic symptoms.

During NAET evaluation, the NAET doctor— before proceeding with the treatments—checks out all these factors. If practiced regularly, it takes only a few seconds to rule out all these unusual factors. A NAET practitioner is well trained to test and determine the influences of emotions in the present health conditions.

If not taken care of, asthma can turn into emphysema, in which the inner lining of the lungs and the air bags (alveoli) lose their elasticity. This makes it hard for the air to go in and out of the lungs freely. Oxygen exchange between the lungs and outside air becomes difficult. In advanced cases, the expanded air bags inside the lungs give the sufferer the appearance of someone with a barrel chest. In the early stages, the patient can get prompt relief with NAET.

INGESTANTS

Ingestants are allergens that are contacted in the normal course of eating a meal or that enter the system in other ways through the mouth and find their way into the gastrointestinal tract. These include: foods, drinks, condiments, drugs, beverages, chewing gums, vitamin supplements, etc. All these are potential allergens that trigger various sensitive reactions any time in sensitive individuals. We must not ignore the potential reactions to things that may be touched and inadvertently transmitted into the mouth by our hands too.

Sulfites are widely publicized substances that have been added as a preservative to salads and potatoes in restaurant salad bars and in the fast food industry. The intention was to maintain freshness (or at least the appearance of freshness and flavor) as these vegetables sit out in display cases for long periods of time. Unfortunately, sulfites are salt derivatives of sulfuric acid, which many chemically sensitive persons are highly allergic to.

The area of ingested allergens is one of the hardest to diagnose, because the allergic responses are often delayed from several minutes to several days, making the direct association between cause and effect very difficult. This is not to say that an immediate response is not possible. Some people can react violently in seconds after they consume the allergens. In extreme cases, one has to only touch or come near the allergen to signal the central nervous system that it is about to be poisoned, resulting in symptoms that are peculiar to that particular patient. Usually, more violent reactions are observed in ingested allergens than in other forms.

Such was the case of Steve, a young man in his early teens, who had come to the office for a sports-related injury. He also had a history of asthma. On one occasion, his mother brought to the doctor's attention that her son had some continuous itching in an area four finger widths below the knee, on the outer side of the anterior tibial crest. The itching was on the stomach meridian, which meant that the cause of the allergic rash was related to something he was eating frequently. On questioning him further, it was revealed that whenever he ate his favorite breakfast cereal he broke out in a rash.

A simple experiment was set up for confirmation of the effect of the cereal. He was given all his breakfast items: juice, toast and rice cereal, one by one. Then he was given time to chew. All went well until he placed one, and only one, rice cereal flake in his mouth and chewed. He immediately complained of feeling hot and began to redden in an allergic rash, and in a few more seconds he had almost slipped into an anaphylactic shock. After several tense minutes and continuous treatment by NAET, his symptoms subsided.

In a similar, but unfortunately more tragic instance, peanuts were responsible for the death of an otherwise healthy 12-year-old boy in Midwestern United States. Although he knew that he was allergic to peanuts, he accidentally ate them as an ingredient in cookies after a Little League game. He died shortly after reaching the hospital in anaphylactic shock.

Literally any substance we eat can become an allergen for someone who is sensitive to any ingredient in the product. For instance, some chemically sensitive people have been known to faint every time they eat an orange, without exhibiting any other food allergies. By avoiding this allergen they can prevent the occurrence of an allergic reaction and may find it unnecessary to subject themselves to regular medical care. However, one should keep in mind that in this and similar minor allergy cases, patients who are not treated tend to manifest allergic symptoms to other similar allergens in the future. For example, a patient who fainted when she ate a banana might develop asthma or migraine headaches when she eats an orange at a later date. She may be allergic to potassium, one of the basic ingredients in the banana and orange.

We live in a highly technological age. New substances are being introduced into our diets that preserve color, flavor and extend the shelf life of our foods. Some additives used in foods as preservatives have caused severe health problems. Some artificial sweeteners cause mysterious problems in some chemically sensitive people and may mimic various serious diseases, such as multiple sclerosis, acute prostatitis, trigeminal neuralgia, vertigo, chronic dry cough, joint pains and sciatica, to name a few. Most of these additives are harmless to most people but can be fatal to some who react to these substances.

Rebecca, a 68-year-old lady, was diagnosed as having "Lupus Erythematosus and arthritis." Her white blood cell count dropped as low as 2,000/cubic millimeter. She was advised to get a blood transfusion. During her initial visit in our office, she said that she had been taking 6 to 8 grams of vitamin C daily for the previous six months. Upon questioning her further, it was discovered that her joint pains had begun six months before and that the blood count drop was discovered only two months ago. She was found to be highly allergic to vitamin C. She was treated for vitamin C. Ten days after she finished the treatment for vitamin C, she was tested for white blood cell count and her count had gone up to 7,000/cm, which was normal.

Janet, 24, came in complaining of bilateral breast abscesses over a period of three days. She had severe pain and could not wear normal clothes due to swelling and pain. She had eaten potatoes four days in a row before she developed the pain and swelling of the breast. She was treated for potato by NAET immediately. She felt 60% better soon after the treatment. She needed two more treatments and at the end of two days her breasts became normal. Amazingly, the body healed itself by disposing of the redness, abscess-filled boils, and the painful abscess.

Cecilia, 36, was introduced to a new, alcoholic cocktail that consisted of grapefruit juice, Irish whiskey and tequila. She drank this cocktail every night for three nights in a row. The fourth morning she woke up with a severe pain in her left ovary. She saw her gynecologist and got the terrible news that she had a large mass in the left ovary. Concerned, the gynecologist sent her for an ultrasound examination. She had an orange sized cyst in the left ovary. She was advised by the group of doctors to have surgery immediately to prevent pain and rupture of the cyst, and sent to the emergency room.

Cecilia was one of our patients who had previously been treated in our office for various allergic reactions. She was surprised by the news of the cyst and the possible surgery. Her husband was away on a business trip. Nervous and frightened, she remembered to call me to ask my opinion about the situation. From the series of questions she answered, the cause of the sudden appearance of the cyst was pinpointed to the alcoholic cocktails she drank three nights in a row.

She was asked to come to our office with the cocktail. She was treated by NAET for the allergy to the drink and was given acupuncture to reduce the pain and discomfort. She complained of nausea, dizziness, and excruciating pain on the left lower quadrant of the abdomen. The acupuncture points and methods used for the treatment were Spleen-6, Pericardium-6, with tonification, Large Intestine-3, bilateral and 'ashi' points with the reduction method. Within 40 minutes of the treatment, her pain was reduced to '1' on a scale of 1 - 10. She was treated everyday with acupuncture for the next three days. Then an ultrasound test was repeated. All of the tests performed on her were negative for any cysts.

Food coloring causes many allergies among people. Young school-going children consume various food colorings in large quantity in various forms: ice cream, candies, chewing gums, etc. Many children suffer from hyperactivity, poor concentration, irritability, autistic behaviors, hives, rashes, itching, eczema, etc. These are expected common symptoms of food colorings. Unusual symptoms like adrenal depletion, profuse sweating after eating food colorings confuse the patients and the physicians.

Homogenized milk causes concern to a lot of patients in the United States. Even after they clear for the milk allergy, homogenized milk drinkers can face some allergic reactions once in a while. This depends mainly on cattle feed. It was found out from various dairies that they have no control over what the cows are fed every day. Most of the nut-oil companies, after extracting the oils, dry the leftovers into compact cakes and sell them to the dairies. In the dairies, these cakes are randomly fed to the cows. When the cows secrete milk, some of the substances from the nuts are also secreted through the milk. Sometimes, if the cows are fed with hay and grasses that are sprayed with pesticides, these substances are also excreted in the milk. In most dairies in different countries it is permitted to add a few drops of chlorox or bleach or formalin (up to 16 drops per gallon) which is added in the milk to prevent contamination or growth of microflora and thus to increase shelf-life. A person who is allergic to this chemical, can react severely while consuming this milk. This particular reaction is not due to any allergy to milk but to the chemical or pesticides or other ingredients in the milk. This should be kept in mind when treating for a milk allergy.

Great care must be taken while testing and treating for these types of foods, because it might help to get a better prognosis when you know what other ingredients are in the product. If everyone could get proficient in muscle-response testing, most hazardous accidents from food allergies could be prevented by testing before consuming the foods.

CONTACTANTS

Contactants produce their effect by direct contact with the skin. They include the well-known poison oak, poison ivy, poison sumac, cats, dogs, rabbits, cosmetics, soaps, skin cremes, detergents, rubbing alcohol, gloves, hair dyes, various types of plant oils, chemicals such as gasoline, dyes, acrylic nails, nail polish, fabrics, formaldehyde, furniture, cabinets, etc.

Allergic reactions to contactants can be different in each person, and may include asthma, eczema, skin rashes, hives, fainting spells, migraine headaches, cough, joint pains, various kinds of arthritis, stomach aches, constipation, mental confusion, swelling of the body, frequent urination, mental irritability, insomnia, skin cancer, etc. It is apparent that something contacted by the skin can produce symptoms as devastating to the patient as anything ingested or inhaled.

John, 38, had suffered from depression for most of his life. He had tried various treatments, including psychotherapy. He was found to be allergic to iron. He had wrought-iron ornamental works all over his house. When he was treated for iron metal, his depression cleared.

Amy, 28, was under treatment for lupus at a lupus clinic. She had severe joint pains most of the time. She suffered from severe insomnia, mental cloudiness, poor memory, mental irritability and debilitating multiple joint pains. She was on three different kinds of analgesics, which she took every three hours, to control her pain. Extremely hot, cold or cloudy weather affected her immensely. On such days, she stayed indoors with pain pills and warm water. When she was evaluated in our office, she was found to be allergic to all the fabrics she was wearing, however, she was not allergic to any food or drugs. She was treated individually for cotton, polyester, acrylic, nylon, plastics and leather. At the end of the session, it was found that her symptoms of lupus had diminished greatly. Her bodily disturbances with the weather changes also disappeared. She had been visiting the lupus clinic once a month. When she visited the clinic after she cleared her allergies, she showed great improvement in her laboratory blood tests. She was told the best news by her doctor — that her lupus was in remission. Six years later, she remains absolutely symptom-free.

Woolen clothes may also cause allergies. We have seen people who cannot wear wool without breaking out in rashes. Some people who are sensitive to wool also react to creams with lanolin base, since lanolin is derived from sheep wool. Some people can be allergic to cotton socks, orlon socks, or woolen socks with symptoms of knee pain, etc. People can also be allergic to carpets and drapes that could cause knee pains and joint pains.

We had a few other female patients who were allergic to their panty hose and suffered from leg cramps, high blood pressure, swollen legs, psoriasis, and persistent yeast infections. Toilet paper and paper towels also cause problems, mimicking yeast infections in many people.

Many people are allergic to underarm deodorants and antiperspirants, causing skin rashes, irritation of the skin, dermatitis, boils, infections, lymph gland swelling and pain. The chemicals in the antiperspirants and deodorants are toxic and carcinogenic to some people. These products do their intended job, that is to prevent sweating, by blocking the sweat glands. That could lead to inflammation of the sweat glands, and constant irritation and inflammation can lead to more chronic disorders like breast cancer.

Many people are allergic to dry cleaning chemicals. Many women are allergic to their synthetic bras and to feminine tampons. There are reports from women-sufferers that probably their allergy to antiperspirant or usage of synthetic bras caused some of them to have fibrocystic breasts, breast lumps, breast cancers, and that tampons might have caused cervical cancer.

Many people are allergic to crude oils and their derivatives, which include plastic and synthetic rubber products. Can you imagine the difficulty of living in this modern society, trying to be completely free from products made of crude oil? A person would literally be immobilized. The phones we use, the naugahyde chairs we sit on, the milk containers we use, the polyester fabrics we wear, most of the face and body creams we use, all are made from a common product - crude oil!

Food items, normally classified as ingestants, may also act as contactants on persons who handle them constantly over time. Cooks who knead the wheat flour daily could suffer from respiratory disorders like asthma, emphysema or even angina or coronary heart diseases. People who cut vegetables and pack them in the grocery stores could suffer from skin rashes and eczema from the allergy to the vitamin C from the vegetables. Some people suffer from fibromyalgia and chronic fatigue by continuous exposure to certain vegetables and food products like cutting and canning peppers or onions.

Other career-produced allergies have been diagnosed for cooks, waiters, grocery-store keepers, clerks, gardeners, etc. Virtually no trade or skill is exempt from contracting allergens.

INJECTANTS

Allergens are injected into the skin, muscles, joints and blood vessels in the form of various serums, antitoxins, vaccines and drugs. As in any other allergic reaction, the injection of a sensitive drug into the system runs the risk of producing dangerous allergic reactions. To the chemically sensitive person, the drug actively becomes a poison, with the same effect as an injection of arsenic. No one would intentionally give an injection of a potentially dangerous drug to a person. However, some drugs seem to become more allergenic for certain people over time, without the person being aware of the potential risk. Take the increasing incidents of allergies to the drug penicillin as an example. The reactions vary in people, from hives to diarrhea to anaphylactic shock and death.

Most of us do not often consider an insect bite in the same way as we would an injection received from a physician or a member of his staff, but the result is quite the same. At the point of the bite, a minute amount of the body fluid (saliva) of the insect is injected into the body. These fluids may be incidental to the bite. They may be simply secretions normal to the salivary gland or biting part of the insect, or they may be a necessary part of the biting mechanism, such as the saliva of the mosquito, which is formulated to keep the host's blood from coagulating so blood extraction is not difficult. These fluids may also be specifically formulated to produce immobilizing pain, in order to protect the insect from its own predators, such as the spider that uses its bite to secure food and inflict pain in the defense of its territory, the bee that uses its sting for defense, and the wasp that uses its sting to obtain food and defend its nest.

Certain animal bites also inject near-lethal amounts of toxins into the bloodstream of victims, again to immobilize the prey and to protect itself from its own predators, and for accidental harm from a clumsy neighbor. Examples include the general classification of pit vipers and one or two lizards. Bites from mammals also fit into this category. They include children's bites which can produce considerable infection at the site of the bite, and the injection of the dreaded virus from the bite of an infected animal.

The normal reaction to a bite, other than the obvious lethal bites, ranges from mild swelling around the site of the injection, a mild reddening and, of course, a slight to moderate discomfort in the body from attempting to free the toxin that produces itching. Rarely are these bites and stings lethal to the normally insensitive person.

For some people, however, a sting or a bite by an animal or insect is potentially lethal. Even a single mosquito bite may produce an extreme and sudden onset of edema (the abnormal collection of fluids in the body tissue and cells) and severe respiratory distress. There have been many cases of anaphylactic shock, respiratory and/or cardiac failure in sensitive persons, following the slightest insect bite.

INFECTANTS

Infectants are allergens that produce their effect by causing a sensitivity to an infectious agent, such as bacteria. For example, when tuberculin bacteria is introduced as part of a diagnostic test to determine a patient's sensitivity and/or reaction to that particular agent, an allergic reaction may result. This may occur during skin patch, or scratch tests done in the normal course of allergy testing in traditional Western medical circles.

Infectants differ from injectants as allergens because of the nature of the allergenic substances; that is, the substance is a known injectant and is limited in the amount administered to the patient. A slight prick of the skin introduces the toxin through the epidermis and a pox or similar harmless skin lesion will erupt if the patient is allergic or reactive to that substance. For most people, the pox soon dries up and forms a scab which eventually drops off, without much discomfort. However, for those individuals who are reactive to these tests, it is not uncommon to experience fainting, nausea, fever, swelling (not only at the scratch site but over the whole body), respiratory distress, etc.

In other words, the introduction of an allergen into the chemically sensitive person's system runs the potential risk of causing a severe reaction, regardless of the reason or the amount of the toxic substance used. Great care must be taken in the administration of tests that are designed to produce an allergic reaction.

Various vaccinations and immunizations may also produce such allergic reactions. Some children after they receive their usual immunization get very sick physically and emotionally.

Many children suffering from attention deficit and hyperactive disorders, learning disability, and autism have returned to normalcy after clearing their allergies through NAET® (The journal of NAET® Energetics and Complementary Medicine, (2)(2), 2006).

It should be noted that bacteria, virus, etc. are contacted in numerous ways. Our casual contact with objects and people exposes us daily to dangerous contaminants and possible illnesses. When our autoimmune systems are functioning properly, we pass off the illness without notice. When our systems are not working at maximum performance levels, we experience infections, fevers, etc.

From a strictly allergenic standpoint, however, contact with an injectant does not produce the expected reaction for that particular injectant; rather a more typical allergic reaction takes place, as can be seen in the tuberculin test as an example. It is clear that the reaction to the test would probably not be a case of tuberculosis but rather a mild allergic response such as an infectious eruption under the skin.

Wanda, 36, had experienced multiple sclerosis for 12 years. Her symptoms began after giving birth by Cesarean section. During the childbirth, she was injected with spinal anesthesia. She was found to be highly allergic to the spinal anesthesia that was used 12 years before. Her symptoms got better when she was cleared for the allergy to the anesthesia.

Julia, 26, was found to have had multiple sclerosis for the previous five years. When she came to our office, she was unable to walk without assistance, and she was almost blind in both eyes. In her case, her silicone breast implant was the cause. When she was cleared for the silicone implant, her symptoms got better. She regained her sight, she became steady on her feet, was able to pass the driver's license test and drive again.

PHYSICAL AGENTS

Heat, cold, sunlight, dampness, drafts or mechanical irritants may also cause allergic reactions and are known as physical allergens. When the patient suffers from more than one allergy, physical agents can affect the patient greatly. If the patient has already eaten some allergic food item, then walks in cold air or drafts, he might develop upper respiratory problems, sore throat, asthma or joint pains, etc., depending on his tendency toward health problems. Some people are very sensitive to cold or heat, whether they have eaten any allergic food or not. Such cases are common.

Helene, 74, liked to drink cold water, but she always choked on icy cold water. She also developed an allergic dry cough whenever she ate ice cream. She was treated for all the ingredients in the ice cream, yet her coughing spells and choking incidents persisted. She was finally treated for actual ice cubes. Afterwards, she could enjoy ice water and ice cream without choking.

Maria, 49, had experienced severe hot flashes for three years. She was on hormone supplements, but nothing gave her relief. She was found to be allergic to heat, sugar and hormones. After she was cleared for the allergy to the above items, her hot flashes stopped completely.

Jenny, 58, suffered from Raynaud's disease. The tip of her fingers remained dark blue on a cold day. She was allergic to cold, citrus fruits, and meat products. She felt better when she was cleared for the above items.

Many arthritic patients, asthma patients, migraine patients, PMS patients, and mental patients have exaggerated symptoms on cold, cloudy or rainy days. These types of patients could suffer from severe allergy to electrolytes, cold, or a combination of both.

Some patients react to heat or cold violently, getting aches and pains during a cloudy day, and icy cold hands and feet even if they are clad in multiple warm socks. These patients have hypofunctioning immune systems. When they finish the treatment program, they do not continue to feel cold or get sick with the heat or cold.

GENETIC CAUSES

Discovery of possible tendencies toward allergies carried over from parents and grandparents opens a large door to achieving optimum health. Most people inherit the allergic tendency from their parents or grandparents. Allergies can also skip generations and be manifested very differently in children.

Many people with various allergic manifestations respond well to the treatment of various disease agents that have been transmitted from parents.

A woman who suffered from bronchial asthma was cleared of her asthma when she was treated for pneumococcus, the bacterium responsible for pneumonia. Both of her parents had died of pneumonia soon after her birth.

Ray, a man of 44, responded well to the treatment for diphtheria, thus clearing his chronic bronchitis. He had inherited the tendency toward allergies from his mother, who almost died from diphtheria when she was seven. The reaction to diphtheria was manifested in him as bronchitis, sinusitis and arthritis.

Jill, 55, suffered from the Epstein-Barr virus and various allergies. After treatment for the virus, her response was very encouraging. Upon questioning her, it was found that her Japanese parents, uncles and aunts died of tuberculosis. She was immediately tested and treated for tuberculosis and she became allergy free and healthy once again.

Parents with rheumatic fever may transmit the disease to their offspring, but in the children the rheumatic fever agent may not be manifested in its original form. As example, Sara, 42, had severe migraines all her life. Her mother had rheumatic fever as a child. Treatment for rheumatic fever lessened her migraines.

MOLDS AND FUNGI

Molds and fungi are in a category by themselves, because of the numerous ways they are contacted as allergens in everyday life. They can be ingested, inhaled, touched or even, as in the case of Penicillin, injected. They come in the form of airborne spores, making up a large part of the dust we breathe or pick up in our vacuum cleaners; fluids such as our drinking water; as dark fungal growth in the corners of damp rooms; as athlete's foot; and in particularly obnoxious vaginal conditions commonly called "yeast infections." They grow on trees and in the damp soil. They are a source of food, as in truffles and mushrooms; of diseases such as ring worm and the aforementioned yeast infections, and of healing, as in the tremendous benefits mankind has derived from the drug Penicillin.

Reactions to these substances are as varied as other kinds of allergies. This is because they are a part of one of the largest known classifications of biological entities. Because of the number of ways they can be introduced into the human anatomy, the number of reactions are multiplied considerably. Fungi are parasites that grow on living as well as decaying organic matter. That means that some forms are found growing in the human anatomy. The problem of athlete's foot is a prime example.

Athlete's foot is a human parasite fungus that grows anywhere in the body, where the area is fairly moist and not exposed to sunlight or air. It is particularly difficult to eliminate, and treatment generally consists of a topical preparation, multiple daily cleansing of the area, a medicinal powder, and wearing light cotton socks to avoid further infection from dyes used in colored wearing apparel.

It is contracted by contact with the fungus and is often passed from person to person anywhere there is the potential for contact (i.e gymnasiums, showers, locker rooms and other areas where people share facilities and walk barefoot), thus the name athlete's foot. If it is a real athlete's foot, it will clear with the

NAET® treatment. Certain allergies, like allergies to socks made of cotton, orlon, or nylon, etc., can mimic athlete's foot. In such cases, athlete's foot may not clear by using medications.

Allergies to cotton, orlon, nylon, or paper could result in the explosions of infections including Ascomycetes fungi (yeast) that women are finding so troublesome. Feminine tampons, toilet papers, douches, and deodorants can also cause yeast infections.

EMOTIONAL STRESSORS

Many times, the origin of physical symptoms can be traced back to some unresolved emotional trauma. Each cell in the body (meridians) has the capability to respond physically, physiologically and psychologically to our daily activities. When the vital energy flows evenly and uninterrupted through the energy pathways (acupuncture meridians), the body functions normally. When there is a disruption in the energy flow through the meridians (an increase or decrease), energy blockages can occur, causing various emotional symptoms in those particular meridians. According to Oriental medical theory, there are seven major emotions which can cause pathological health problems in people: sadness affects lung meridian, joy affects the heart, disgust affects the stomach, anger affects the liver, worry affects the spleen, fear affects the kidney, and depression affects the pericardium meridian. Please read chapter 5 for more information.

IRRITATION AND FATIGUE FROM EATING
PRODUCTS WITH SUGAR

Dear Dr. Devi,

I want to relate to you my experience with the NAET® emotional treatment. I was a student in the NAET® advanced level 1 class this past December. To demonstrate an NAET® emotional treatment you called for a volunteer and I submitted myself as a Guinea pig. In muscle testing me you found that I was reactive to sugar at my emotional level and began inquiring of my body when this allergy began. I had noticed that whenever I ate sugar, I used to get irritable and later fatigued. You found that at sometime around the age of 21 or 22, I had an experience with a man I loved that caused me to become allergic to sugar. I could not remember the event, try as I might, but you were able to do the treatment without my recalling the full memory of the event.

A short time later, the class took a break for a delicious lunch of vegetarian food. As I was finishing my meal I suddenly remembered the incident that caused me much pain which fitted all the criteria that you had discovered in the muscle testing. When I was about 22 years old I was a professional singer and working with a group in another city. During this gig I fell in love with the keyboard player and we began an affair. A month later I left the band, as previously arranged, as I was retiring from club work. He and I stayed in touch by phone and planned to continue our relationship when he returned to Los Angeles.

A few weeks after my return home, my paramour was having a birthday and I decided to surprise him with a visit. I ordered a cake with special decorations and carefully transported it to its destination by hand. When I arrived at his door, my greeting was much less than a joyful reunion I had expected; he looked shocked and a bit sheepish. When he recovered his composure he seemed himself again but the damage was done and I felt unwelcome. As the weekend progressed it became clear that he'd picked up where we had left off with my replacement, the new girl singer that I had trained. Needless to say, the rest of the weekend was a disaster.

That was a very painful time in my life and the experience left me with an emotional allergy to sugar which remained undiscovered until you tested and treated me in the class. Sugar consumption doesn't make me tired or irritable anymore. I now have no unpleasant emotions when I recall this incident, proof enough for me that you can unlock secrets of our psyches and treat the effects of emotional trauma with NAET®.

Karen HA, OMD, L.Ac.

3

Detecting Allergies

Allergic conditions occur much more frequently than most people realize. Every year there are more and more recognized cases of allergies in the United States. Statistics show that at least 50 percent of the population suffers from some form of allergy. Many people are interested in understanding the differences and/or the similarities of the methods of diagnosis, the effectiveness and length of treatment between traditional Western medicine and Oriental medicine. Since the purpose of this book is to provide information about the new treatment method of NAET, more attention will be given to Oriental medicine.

With NAET®, it is extremely important for the patient to cooperate with the physician in order to obtain the best results. It is my hope that this chapter will help bring about a clearer understanding between allergists and their patients because, in order to obtain the most satisfactory results, both parties must work together as a team.

Freedom From Chemical Sensitivities

The first step in diagnosing a chemical sensitivity is to take a thorough patient history, including chief complaint, present history, past medical history, family history, social history, history of activities, hobbies and nutrition. It will be beneficial to obtain a thorough record of any past sensitivity reactions in the patient's family, tracing back two or three generations if possible. The patient will be asked whether either parent suffers from asthma or hay fever, ever suffered from hives, reacted to a serum injection (such as tetanus antitoxin, DPT), or experienced any type of skin trouble. Additionally, the allergist will ask whether the patient's parents were unable to eat certain foods or professed to "hate" certain foods because of how the particular food made them feel; complained of sinusitis, runny nose, frequent colds or flu; had dyspepsia, indigestion, mental illness, heart disorders, skin disorders, or any other conditions where an allergy may have been a contributing factor, whether or not recognized as such at the time.

The same questions are asked about the patient's other relatives: grandparents, aunts, uncles, brothers, sisters and cousins. An allergic tendency is not always inherited directly from the parents. It may skip generations, and manifest in nieces or nephews rather than in direct descendants.

The careful allergist will also determine whether such diseases as tuberculosis, cancer, diabetes, rheumatic or glandular disorders exist or have ever occurred in the patient's family history. All of these facts help give the allergist a more complete picture of the hereditary characteristics of the patient. *Allergic tendency* is inherited. It may be manifested differently in different people. Unlike the tendency, an actual allergic condition, such as chemical sensitivity is not always inherited. Parents may have had cancer or rheumatism, but the child can manifest that allergic inheritance as general body ache or chronic fatigue symptoms.

When the family history is complete, the allergist will need to look into the history of the patient's recent history of chemical sensitivity reactions. Some typical preliminary questions include: When did your first episode occur? Did your allergy first occur when you were an infant or a child, or did you first notice the symptoms after you were fully grown? Did it occur after going through a certain procedure? For example, did it occur for the first time after a dental procedure like a root canal? One of my patients reported that her asthma occurred for the first time four hours after root canal work. She was allergic to *Gutta Percha Tissue* that was used in the procedure.

Once a careful history is taken, the allergist often discovers that the patient's first symptoms occurred in early childhood. He or she may have suffered from infantile eczema, but never associated it with asthma which may not have appeared until middle age.

Next, the doctor will want to know the circumstances surrounding and immediately preceding the first symptoms. Typical questions will include: Did you change your diet or go on a special diet? Did you eat something that you hadn't eaten perhaps for two or three months? Do you eat one type of food repeatedly, every day? Did the symptoms follow a childhood illness (whooping cough, measles, chicken pox, diphtheria) or any immunization for such an illness? Did they follow some other illness, such as influenza, pneumonia, viral infection, or a major operation? Did the symptoms first appear at adolescence or after you had a baby? Were they first noticed after you acquired a cat, a dog, or even a bird? Did they appear after an automobile accident or any major physical or mental trauma? Did they appear after a lengthy exposure to the sun, a day at the beach or 18 holes of golf? Did they appear after receiving a gift for your birthday? Or after starting to use a new pair of socks, pants, shirt, after-shave, wrist watch, leather belt, leather shoes, a chair, furniture, certain shampoo, cosmetics? Did your symptoms begin after a new arrival in the house (a baby, a guest, a pet, etc.)?

Any one of these factors can be responsible for triggering a severe allergic manifestation or precipitate the first noticeable symptoms of an allergic condition. Therefore, it is very important to obtain full and accurate answers when taking a patient's medical history.

Other important questions also should relate to the frequency and occurrence of the sensitivity reaction-episodes. Although foods may be a factor, if the symptoms occur only at specific times of the year, the trouble is most likely due to pollens. Often a patient is sensitive to certain foods but has a natural tolerance that prevents sickness until the pollen sensitivity adds sufficient allergens to throw the body into an imbalance. If symptoms occur only on specific days of the week, they are probably due to something contacted or eaten on that particular day.

The causes of allergic attacks in different patients can, at first, appear to be random. Regular weekly attacks of sneezing and nasal allergy were the effects in one patient after he read the Sunday newspaper. The ink caused a severe allergic reaction. Another patient reacted similarly to the comic section of the newspaper. A man always had a gastrointestinal allergic attack on Sunday morning. The cause was traced to eating a traditional pizza every Saturday night with his family. He was allergic to the tomato sauce on the pizza. Still another patient had an allergic attack of sneezing and runny nose on Saturdays. I traced the allergy to the chemical compounds in a lotion she used to set her hair on Friday afternoons.

The time of day when the episodes occur is also of importance in determining the cause of an allergic manifestation. If it always occurs at night, it is quite likely that there is something in the bedroom that is aggravating the condition. It may be that the patient is sensitive to feathers in the pillow or comforter, wood cabinets, marble floors, carpets, side tables, end tables, bed sheets, pillows, pillow cases, detergents used in washing clothes, indoor plants, or shrubs, trees or grasses outside the patient's window.

Many patients react violently to house dust, different types of furniture, polishes, house plants, tap water and purified water. Most city water suppliers change the water chemicals once or twice a year. This is done with good intentions: people with chemical allergies may get sicker if they ingest the same chemicals over and over for months or years. Changing chemicals like chlorine to chloramine and back to chlorine every six months gives an opportunity for the chemically sensitive person not to be continuously exposed to the same chemical throughout the year.

Contrary to traditional Western thinking, developing immunity can be the exception rather than the rule.

Occasionally, switching foods, chemicals or other substances gives a change of allergens to an allergic patient and a chance for him/her to recover from reactions. In this way, some allergies can be avoided.

The doctor should ask the patient to make a daily log of all the foods he/she is eating and all other daily activities. The ingredients in the food should be checked for possible allergens. Certain common allergens like corn products, MSG (monosodium glutamate or Accent), citric acid, etc., are used in many food preparations.

Allergy to corn is one of today's most common allergies, especially in chemically sensitive patients. Unfortunately, corn-starch is found in almost every processed food and some toiletries and drugs as well. Chinese food, baking soda, baking powder and toothpaste contain large amounts of cornstarch. It is the binding product in almost all vitamins and pills, including aspirin and Tylenol. Corn syrup is the natural sweetener in many of the products we ingest, including soft drinks. Corn silk is found in cosmetics and corn oil is used as a vegetable oil. Cotton crotches of female underpants are treated with baking soda and baking powder for better hygiene. But an allergy to corn from baking soda is found to be one of the common sources of never-ending yeast-like infections in chemically sensitive women. Many women became free of yeast-like infections after treating for cornstarch with NAET®.

People react severely to various gums used in many preparations: Acacia gum, xanthine gum, karaya gum, etc. Numerous gums are used in candy bars, yogurt, cream cheese, soft drinks, soy sauce, barbecue sauce, fast food products, macaroni and cheese, etc.

Exposure to any of these items can produce debilitating symptoms in chemically sensitive people. Some of these symptoms are also listed in the pages 53-54.

Very often these symptoms are diagnosed at their face value and the original cause of chemical sensitivity is over looked.

FOOD CHEMICALS

A number of food chemicals are encountered in the food industry and chemically sensitive person has a difficult time when they consume ready-made and packaged foods with these chemicals. A few such food chemicals are: Acetic Acid, Agar, Albumin, Aldicarb, Alginates, Propylene glycol, Aluminum Salts, Sodium aluminum phosphate, Benzoates, Cal. Proprionate, Cal. Silicate, Carbamates, Carbon Monoxide, EDTA, Ethylene gas, Food Bleach, Formic Acid, Malic Acid, Mannan, Mannitol, Salicylic Acid, Succinic Acid, Talc, Tartaric Acid and various water pollutants.

Acetic Acid (sodium acetate and sodium diacetate). This is a common food additive. This is the acid of vinegar. Acetic acid is used as an acidic flavoring agent for pickles, sauces, catsups, mayonnaise, wine, foods that are preserved in vinegar, some soft drinks, processed cheese, baked goods, cheese spreads, sweet and sour drinks and soups. It is also naturally found in apples, cocoa, coffee, wine, cheese, grapes, and other over-ripened fruits. If you get allergic reaction to these natural foods you may be allergic to acetic acid.

Agar (Seaweed extract): This is a polysaccharide that comes from several varieties of algae and it can turn like a gel if you dissolve it in water. So this is used in ice cream, jellies, preserves, icings, laxatives, used as a thickening agent in milk, cream, and used as gelatin (vegetable form). This is a safe additive, but if you are allergic to sea foods you may need to eliminate the allergy for this.

Albumin (cow milk-albumin): Many people are allergic to albumin in the milk. Researchers have found children/people who are allergic to milk albumin are at high risk to get any of these disorders: ADD, ADHD, Autism, bipolar diseases, schizophrenia, and other allergy-related brain disorders. NAET® can desensitize you for milk-albumin.

Aldicarb: It is an organic chemical water pollutant, seen often in city water. When the concentration of this chemical gets high in the city water, many people get sick with gastrointestinal disorders, like nausea, vomiting, pain, bloating, stomach flu, etc. Boiling the water for 30 minutes could help reduce the reaction. If you are not allergic to apple cider vinegar, adding two-three drops of vinegar in eight ounces of water might help.

Alginates (Alginic acid, algin gum, ammonium, calcium, potassium, and sodium alginates, propylene glycol alginates): Most of these are natural extracts of seaweed and used in the food industry primarily as stabilizing agents.

Propylene glycol is an antifreeze. This is supposed to be a safe solvent, used in food preparation, especially in ice creams. Alginates help to retain water. It helps to prevent ice crystal formation; helps uniform distribution of flavors through foods. They add smoothness and texture to the products and are used in ice creams, custards, chocolates, chocolate milk, cheese, salad dressings, jellies, confections, cakes, icings, jams, and some beverages.

Aluminum Salts (alum hydroxide, alum potassium sulfate, sodium alum phosphate, alum ammonium sulfate, and alum calcium silicate).: Aluminum salts are used as a buffer in various products. This helps to balance the acidity. Used as an astringent to keep canned produce firm, to lighten food texture, and used as an anti-caking agent.

Sodium aluminum phosphate is used in baking powder and in self-rising flours. Alum is used as a clarifier for sugar and as a hardening agent. Aluminum hydroxide is used as a leavening agent in baked goods. It is a strong alkali agent that can be toxic but when used in small amounts it is fairly safe. It is also used in antiperspirants and antacids. Aluminum ammonium sulfate is used as an astringent, and neutralizing agent in baking powder and cereals. It can cause burning sensation to the mucous membranes. Overuse of aluminum products may lead to aluminum toxicity and it can affect the brain chemistry. Other sources of aluminum are cookware, deodorants, antacids, aluminum foils, cans and containers.

Benzoates (sodium benzoate).: Benzoic acid occurs naturally in anise, berries, black olive, blueberries, broccoli, cauliflower, cherry bark, cinnamon, cloves, cranberries, ginger, green grapes, green peas, licorice, plums, prunes, spinach, and tea. Benzoic acid or sodium benzoate is commonly used as a preservative in food processing. This is used as a flavoring agent in chocolate, orange, lemon, nut, and other flavors in beverages, baked products, candies, ice creams, and chewing gums and also used as a preservative in soft drinks, margarine, jellies, juices, pickles, and condiments.

This is also used in perfumes and cosmetics to prevent spoilage by microorganisms. Benzoic acid is a mild antifungal agent. It is metabolized by the liver. Large amount of benzoic acid or benzoates can cause intestinal disturbances, can irritate the eyes, skin, and mucous membranes. This causes eczema, acne and other skin conditions in sensitive people.

Cal. Proprionate: (sodium proprionate and proprionic acid): These are found in dairy products, cheese, breads, cakes, baked goods and chocolate products, They are used as preservatives and mold inhibitors. They reduce the growth of molds and some bacteria.

Source: Baked products, breads, rolls, cakes, cup cakes, processed cheese, chocolate products, preserves, jellies, and butter.

Cal. Silicate: Used as an anticaking agent in products, table salt and other foods preserved in powder form used as a moisture control agent.

Carbamates: These pesticides are used widely in many places. Their toxicity is slightly less than some other pesticides like organochlorines. They are known to produce birth defects.

Source: pesticide-sprayed foods.

Carbon Monoxide: CO is an odorless, colorless gas that competes with oxygen for hemoglobin. The affinity of CO for hemoglobin is more than 200-fold greater than that of oxygen. CO causes tissue hypoxia. Headache is one of the first symptoms, followed by confusion, decreased visual acuity, tachycardia, syncope, metabolic acidosis, retinal hemorrhage, coma, convulsions, and death.

Source: Driving through heavy traffic, damaged gas range, leaky valves of the gas line, exhaust pipes, living in a closed up room for long time, trapped firewood smoke, smoke inhalation from being in a closed, running car, an automobile kept running in closed garage for hours, exhaust from autos and other machinery, etc.

Casein: Milk protein. Also used in prepared foods, candies, protein shakes, etc.

EDTA: This is a very efficient polydentate chelator of many divalent or trivalent cations including calcium. This is used primarily in lead poisoning. This is toxic to the kidneys. Adequate hydration is necessary when you take this in any form.

Ethylene gas (used on fruits, especially on green bananas).

Food Bleach: Most of these are used in bleaching the flour products. Benzoil peroxides, chlorine dioxides, nitrosyl chlorides, potassium bromate, mineral salts, potassium iodate, ammonium sulfate, ammonium phosphate, are the most commonly used food bleaches. They whiten the flour. They also improve the appearance. Whatever they are using should be listed on the labels. Sometimes more than one item is used for better benefit.

Formic Acid: This is a caustic, colorless, forming liquid. Naturally seen in ants (ant bite), synthetically produced and used in tanning and dyeing solutions, fumigants and insecticides. This is also used as an artificial flavoring in food preparations.

Malic Acid: A colorless, highly water soluble, crystalline substance, having a pleasant sour taste, and found in apples, grapes, rhubarb, and cactus. This substance is found to be very effective in reducing general body aches. If you are allergic to it, then you can get severe body ache.

Mannan: Polysaccharides of mannose, found in various legumes and in nuts. Allergy to this factor in dried beans causes fibromyalgia-like symptoms in sensitive people.

Mannitol: It is hexahydric alcohol, used in renal function testing to measure glomerular filtration. Used intravenously as an osmotic diuretic.

Salicylic Acid: Amyl, phenyl, benzyl, and methyl salicylates.

A number of foods including almonds, apples, apricots, berries, plums, cloves, cucumbers, prunes, raisins, tomatoes, and wintergreen. Salicylic acid made synthetically by heating phenol with carbon dioxide is the basis of acetyl salicylic acid. Salicylates are also used in a variety of flavorings such as strawberry, root beer, spice, sarsaparilla, walnut, grapes, and mint.

Succinic Acid: Found in meats, cheese, fungi, and many vegetables with its distinct tart, acid taste.

Source: asparagus, broccoli, beets, and rhubarb.

Talc (magnesium silicate): Talc is a silica chalk that is used in coating, polishing rice and as an anticaking agent. It is used externally on the body surface to dry the area. Talc is thought to be carcinogenic. It may contain asbestos particles. White rice is polished and coated with it.

Tartaric Acid: This is a flavor enhancer. It is a stabilizer.

Commonly seen Water Chemicals (in drinking water).

Alum sulfate, ammonium chloride, benzene, carbon tetrachloride, chlorine, DDT, ferric chloride, gasoline, heavy metals (mercury, silver, zinc, arsenic, lead, copper), organochlorides, organophosphates, PCBs, pesticides, petroleum products, Sodium hydroxide, toluene, and xylene.

Commonly seen Water pollutants: There are many water pollutants we see in our water. Some of them get filtered out by the time we receive in our tap. Most of these pollutants still remain in small amounts. Some of these are inorganic water pollutants like: arsenic, asbestos, cadmium, chromium, copper, cyanide, Lead, mercury, nickels, nitrates, nitrosamines, selenium, silica, silver, and zinc.

Organic chemical water pollutants: 1,2, dichloroethane, 2,4,5,T, 2,4,-D., aldicarb, benzene, carbon tetrachloride, chloroform, DDT, dibromo-chloropropane (DBCP), dichlorobenzene, dioxane, endrin, ethylene dibromide (EDB), gasoline, lindane, methoxychlor, polychlorinated biphenyls (PCB), polynuclear aromatic hydrocarbon (PAH), tetrachloroethylene, toluene, toxaphene, trichloromethane, trichloroethylene (TCE), vinyl chloride, MTBE (Methyl tertiary butyl ether is a gasoline additive), and xylene.

As I have stated earlier, in my opinion, the people who get labelled with various health disorders may be suffering from simple undiagnosed allergies. Many food, chemical and environmental allergic symptoms overlap or mimic a variety of diseases including many neurological and brain disorders.

After completing the patient's history, the NAET specialist should examine the patient for the usual vital signs. A physical examination is performed to check for any abnormal growth or condition. If the patient has an area of discomfort in the body, it should be inspected. It is important to note the type and area of discomfort and its relationship to an acupuncture point. Most pain and discomfort in the body usually occurs around some important acupuncture point.

NAMBUDRIPAD'S TESTING TECHNIQUES (NTT)

NAET uses many standard allopathic and kinesiological testing procedures to detect allergies. Some of the common ones are mentioned below.

1. HISTORY

A complete history of the patient is taken. A symptom survey form is given to the patient to record the level and type of discomfort he/she is suffering.

2. PHYSICAL EXAMINATION

Observation of the mental status, face, skin, eyes, color, posture, movements, gait, tongue, scars, wounds, marks, body secretions, etc.

3. VITAL SIGNS

Evaluation of blood pressure, pulse, skin temperature and palpable pains in the course of meridians, etc.

4. SRT (ELECTRO-DERMAL TEST-EDT)

Skin Resistance Test for the presence or absence of a suspected allergen is done through a computerized electrodermal testing device; differences in the meter reading are observed (the greater the difference, the stronger the allergy).

5. NST

Neuromuscular sensitivity testing (aka muscle response testing) is conducted to compare the strength of a predetermined muscle in the presence and absence of a suspected allergen. If the particular muscle (test muscle) weakens in the presence of an item, it signifies that the item is an allergen. If the muscle remains strong, the substance is not an allergen. More explanation on NST will be given in Chapter 5.

6. DYNAMOMETER TESTING

A hand-held dynamometer is used to measure finger strength

(0-100 scale) in the presence and absence of a suspected allergen. The dynamometer is held with thumb and index finger and squeezed to make the reading needle swing between 0-100 scale. An initial base-line reading is observed first, then the allergen is held and another reading taken. The finger strength is compared in the presence of the allergen. If the second reading is more than the initial reading, there is no allergy. If the second reading is less than the initial reading, then there is an allergy.

7. EMF TEST (ELECTRO MAGNETIC FIELD TEST)

The electromagnetic component of the human energy field can be detected with simple muscle response testing. The pool of electromagnetic energy around an object or a person allows the energy exchange. The human field absorbs the energy from the nearby object and processes it through the network of nerve energy pathways. If the foreign energy field shares suitable charges with the human energy field, the human field absorbs the foreign energy for its advantage and becomes stronger. If the foreign energy field carries unsuitable charges, the human energy field causes repulsion of the foreign energy field. These types of reactions of the human field can be determined by testing an indicator muscle (specific muscle) before and after coming in contact with an allergen.

8. PULSE TEST

Pulse testing is another simple way of determining food allergy. This test was developed by Arthur Coca, M.D. in the 1950's. Research has shown that if you are allergic to something and you eat it, your pulse rate speeds up.

Step 1: Establish your base-line pulse by counting radial pulse at the wrist for a full minute.

Step 2: Put a small portion of the suspected allergen in the mouth, preferably under the tongue. Taste the substance for two minutes. Do not swallow any portion of it. The taste will send the signal to the brain, which will send a signal through the sympathetic nervous system to the rest of the body.

Step 3: Retake the pulse with the allergen still in the mouth. An increase or decrease in pulse rate of 10% or more is considered an allergic reaction. The greater the degree of allergy, the greater the difference in the pulse rate. This test is useful to test food allergies. If you are allergic to very many foods, and if you consume a few allergens at the same time, it will be hard to detect the exact allergen causing the reaction just by this test.

9. NAET ROTATION DIET

After clearing the allergy to the basic NAET allergens, the foods from the allergy-free list is consumed in a pre-selected order. Then use the question response test (ask questions while doing NST and the muscle weakness will be interpreted as "yes" answer, and a muscle strength will be interpreted as "no" answer. Every meal is selected from a non-allergic list according to the priority. This prevents overload of the particular food in the body and reduces unwanted allergic reactions and allergy-based disorders.

10. HOLD, SIT AND TEST

This is a simple procedure to test allergies. Place a small portion of the suspected allergen in a baby food jar or thin-glass jar, preferably with a lid, then the person will hold it in her/his palm, touching the jar with the fingertips of the same hand for 15 to 30 minutes. If the person is allergic to the item in the jar, he/she will begin to feel uneasy when holding the allergen in the palm, giving rise to various unpleasant symptoms. This testing procedure is described in detail in Chapter 6. When we treat patients who have a history of anaphylaxis to a particular item, we use this method after completing the required NAET treatments and before the patient begins to use the item again.

If the patient was treated for a severe peanut allergy, (or milk, egg, wheat, fish, mushroom, etc.) after going through the required NAET treatments to neutralize the peanut, the patient is allowed to sit and hold the peanuts in a glass jar every day for 30 minutes for three days to a week. If the patient does not show any symptoms of previous allergy, he/she will be allowed to hold a peanut in the hand without a bottle for three to five days, 30 minutes daily. If that does not produce any allergic reaction, then the patient will be allowed to put a small piece of nut in the mouth and hold it there for five to ten minutes every day for a few days. If that also does not produce any reaction, the patient will be allowed to eat a small piece of the nut and observe the reaction. Usually, by this time, the patient will be able to use the allergen confidently without fear. Check with your practitioner for more details.

11. ELISA/ACT

ELISA/ACT is distinctive in identifying reactions to all delayed or hidden immune reactions. This includes antibodies (functionally significant IgA, IgM, and IgG) as well as immune complexes and cell-mediated responses. Only a cell culture of all relevant lymphocyte (white cells with long life in circulation) types can give this information. ELISA/ACT is a highly sensitive cell response test which provides a specific fingerprint for each person by identifying substances, typically 6-20 items out of up to 340 that can be tested.

12. SCRATCH TEST

Western medical allergists generally depend on skin testing (scratch test, patch test, etc.), in which a very small amount of a suspected allergic substance is introduced into the person's skin through a scratch or an injection. The site of injection is observed for any reaction. If there is any reaction at the area of injection, the person is considered to be allergic to that substance. Each item has to be tested individually.

13. RADIOALLERGOSORBANT TEST (RAST)

The RAST measures IgE antibodies in serum and identifies specific allergens causing allergic reactions.

14. ELIMINATION DIET

The elimination diet, which was developed by Dr. Albert H. Rowe of Oakland, California, consists of a very limited diet that must be followed for a period long enough to determine whether or not any of the foods included in it are responsible for the allergic symptoms. The importance of adhering strictly to the diet during the diagnostic period is very crucial.

4

Symptoms of Meridians

An allergy means an altered reactivity. Reactions and aftereffects can be measured using various standard medical diagnostic tests. Energy medicine has also developed various devices to measure the reactions. Oriental medicine has used "Medical I Ching" since 3,322 BC. Another simple way to test one's body is through simple, kinesiological neuromuscular sensitivity testing (NST) procedures (Chapter 5). It is an easy procedure for a person to evaluate his/her progress.

Study of the acupuncture meridians is helpful to understand NST and how it works. All living beings have energy meridians and nerve energy circulates through these meridians throughout the day and night. If one learns to identify abnormal symptoms connected with acupuncture meridians, detection of the causative agents (allergens) will be easier. The true functions and pathological functions of the twelve major acupuncture meridians are described in the next few pages.

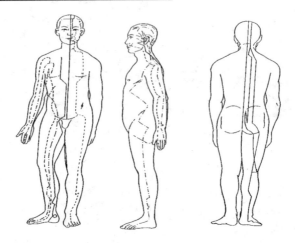

ENERGY FLOW THROUGH 12 MERIDIANS
FIGURE 4-1

NORMAL ENERGY FLOW

Lung--> Large Intestine--> Stomach-->Spleen--> Heart--> Small Intestine-->Urinary Bladder--> Kidney--> Pericardium-->Triple Warmer--> Gall Bladder--> Liver-->Lung

THE LUNG MERIDIAN (LU)

Energy disturbance in the lung meridian affecting physical and physiological levels can give rise to the following symptoms:

Asthma between 3-5 a.m.
Atopic dermatitis
Bronchiectasis
Bronchitis
Burning in the eyes, & nostrils
Cardiac asthma
Chest congestion & cough
Coughing up blood
Cradle cap
Dry mouth, skin, throat
Emaciated look
Emphysema
Fever with chills
Frequent flu-like symptoms
General body ache with burning sensation
Generalized hives
Hair loss
Hair thinning
Hay-fever
Headache between eyes
Inability to sleep after 3 a.m.
Infantile eczema
Infection in the respiratory tract
Itching of the body, scalp, nose
Lack of desire to talk
Lack or excessive of perspiration
Laryngitis and pharyngitis
Low voice
Moles
Morning fatigue
Mucus in the throat
Nasal congestion or runny nose

Night sweats
Nose bleed
Pain between third and fourth thoracic vertebrae
Pain in the chest and intercostal muscles
Pain in the eyes
Pain in the first interphalangeal joint and thumb
Pain in the upper arms and back
Pain in the upper first and second cuspids (tooth)
Pleurisy
Pneumonia
Poor growth of nails and hair
Postnasal drip
Red cheeks and eyes
Restlessness between 3 to 5 a.m.
Scaly and rough skin
Sinus headaches and infection
Skin rashes
Skin tags
Sneezing
Sore throat
Stuffy nose
Swollen cervical glands
Swollen throat
Tenosynovitis
Thick yellow discharge in case of bacterial infection
Thin or thick white discharge in case of viral infection

Freedom From Chemical Sensitivities

Energy disturbance in the lung meridian affecting the cellular level. When one fails to cry, when one feels deep sorrow, sadness will settle in the lungs and eventually cause various lung disorders

Apologizing
Comparing self with others
Contempt
Dejection
Depression
Despair
False pride
Grief or sadness.
Highly sensitive emotionally
Hopelessness
Intolerance

Likes to humiliate others
Loneliness
Low self-esteem
Meanness
Melancholy
Over demanding
Over sympathy
Prejudice
Seeking approval from others
Self pity
Weeping Frequently

Essential Nutrients to Strengthen the Lung Meridian

Clear water
Proteins
Vitamin A
Vitamin C
Bioflavonoid
Cinnamon
Essential fatty acids
Onions
Garlic

B-vitamins (especially B_2)
Citrus fruits
Green peppers
Black peppers
Rice

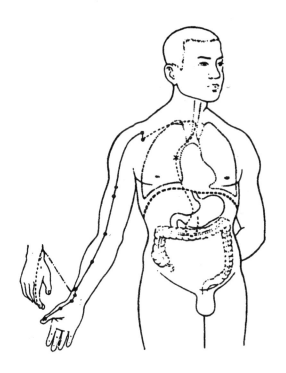

FIGURE 4-1

THE LUNG MERIDIAN (LU)

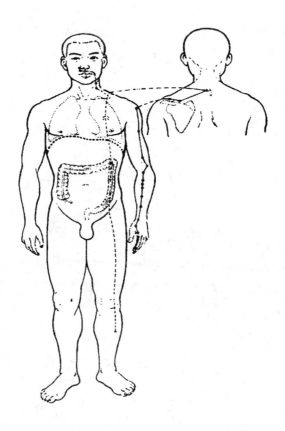

FIGURE 4-2

THE LARGE INTESTINE MERIDIAN (LI)

THE LARGE INTESTINE MERIDIAN (LI)

Energy disturbance in the large intestine meridian affecting physical and physiological levels can give rise to the following symptoms:

Abdominal pain
Acne on the face, sides of
    the mouth and nose
Asthma after 5 a.m.
Arthritis of the shoulder
    joint
Arthritis of the knee joint
Arthritis of the index
    finger
Arthritis of the wrist joint
Arthritis of the lateral part
    of the elbow and hip
Bad breath
Blisters in the lower gum
Bursitis
Dermatitis
Dry mouth and thirst
Eczema
Fatigue
Feeling better after a
    bowel movement
Feeling tired after a bowel
    movement
Flatulence
Inflammation of lower
    gum

Intestinal colic
Itching of the body
Loose stools or constipation
Lower backache
Headaches
Muscle spasms and pain of
lateral aspect of thigh, knee
    and below knee.
Motor impairment of the
fingers
 Pain in the knee
Pain in the shoulder,
    shoulder blade and back of
      the neck
Pain and swelling of the
    index finger
Pain in the heel
Sciatic pain
Swollen cervical glands
Skin rashes
Skin tags
Sinusitis
Tenosynovitis
Tennis elbow
Toothache
Warts on the skin.

Freedom From Chemical Sensitivities

Energy disturbance in the large intestine meridian affecting the cellular level can cause the following:

Guilt

Confusion

Brain fog

Bad dreams

Dwelling on past memory

Crying spells

Defensiveness

Inability to recall dreams

Nightmares

Nostalgia

Rolling restlessly in sleep

Seeking sympathy

Talking in the sleep and Weeping

Essential Nutrients to Strengthen the Large Intestine Meridian

Vitamins A, D, E, C, B, especially B_1, wheat, wheat bran, oat bran, yogurt, and roughage.

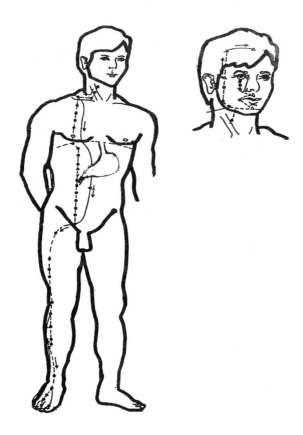

FIGURE 4-3

STOMACH MERIDIAN (ST)

THE STOMACH MERIDIAN (ST)

Energy disturbance in the stomach meridian affecting physical and physiological levels can give rise to the following symptoms:

Abdominal Pains & distention
Acid reflux disorders
Acne on the face and neck
ADD & ADHD
Anorexia
Autism
Bad breath
Black/ blue marks on the
   leg below the knee
Bipolar disorders
Blemishes
Bulimia
Chest muscle pain
Coated tongue
Coldness in the lower limbs
Cold sores in the mouth
Delirium
Depression
Dry nostrils
Dyslexia
Excessive hunger
Facial paralysis
Fever blisters
Fibromyalgia
Flushed face
Frontal headache
Herpes

Heat boils (painful acne) in
the upper front of the body
Hiatal hernia
High fever
Learning disability
Insomnia due to nervousness
Itching on the skin & rashes
Migraine headaches
Manic depressive disorders
Nasal polyps
Nausea
Nosebleed
Pain on the upper jaws
Pain in the mid-back
Pain in the eye
Seizures
Sensitivity to cold
Sore throat
Sores on the gums & tongue
Sweating
Swelling on the neck
Temporomandibular joint
   problem
Unable to relax the mind
Upper gum diseases
Vomiting

Energy disturbance in the stomach meridian affecting the cellular level can cause the following:

Disgust
Bitterness
Aggressive behaviors

Attention deficit disorders
Butterfly sensation in the
stomach

Essential Nutrients to Strengthen the Stomach Meridian

B complex vitamins especially B_{12}, B_6, B_3 and folic acid.

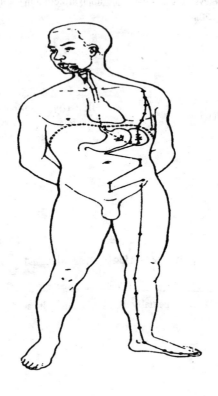

FIGURE 4-4

THE SPLEEN MERIDIAN (SP)

THE SPLEEN MERIDIAN (SP)

Energy disturbance in the spleen meridian affecting physical and physiological levels can give rise to the following symptoms:

Abnormal smell
Abnormal taste
Abnormal uterine bleeding
Absence of menstruation
Alzheimer's disease
Autism
Bitter taste in the mouth
Bleeding from the mucous
    membrane
Bleeding under the skin
Bruises under the skin
Carpal tunnel syndrome
Chronic gastroenteritis
Cold sores on the lips
Coldness of the legs
Cramps after the first day of
    menses
Depression
Diabetes
Dizzy spells
Dreams that make you tired
Emaciated muscles
Failing memory
Fatigue in general
Fatigue of the mind
Fatigued limbs
Feverishness
Fibromyalgia
Fingers and hands-numbness
Fluttering of the eyelids
Frequent
Generalized edema
Hard lumps in the abdomen
Hemophilia

Hemorrhoids
Hyperglycemia
Hypertension
Hypoglycemia
Inability to make decisions
Incontinence of urine or stool
Indigestion
Infertility
Insomnia: usually unable to fall
asleep
Intractable pain anywhere in the
body
Intuitive and prophetic behaviors
Irregular periods
Lack of enthusiasm
Lack of interest in anything
Lethargy
Light-headedness
Loose stools
Nausea
Obesity
Pain and stiffness of the fingers
Pain in the great toes
Pallor
Pedal edema
Pencil-like thin stools with
undigested food particles
Poor memory
Prolapse of the bladder
Prolapse of the uterus
Purpura
Reduced appetite
Sand-like feeling in the eyes
Scanty menstrual flow

Freedom From Chemical Sensitivities

Sensation of heaviness in the
body and head
Sleep during the day
Slowing of the mind
Sluggishness
Schizophrenia
Stiffness of the tongue
Sugar craving
Swelling anywhere in the body
Swellings or pain with swelling
of the toes and feet

Swollen eyelids
Swollen lips
Tingling or abnormal sensation
in the tip of the fingers and
palms
Varicose veins
Vomiting
Watery eyes

Energy disturbance in the spleen meridian affecting the cellular level can cause
the following:

Anxiety
Concern
Does not like crowds
Easily hurt
Gives more importance to self
Hopelessness
Irritable
Keeps feelings inside
Lack of confidence
Likes loneliness
Likes to be praised
Likes to take revenge

Lives through others
Low self esteem
Needs constant encouragement
Obsessive compulsive
behavior
Over sympathetic to others
Unable to make decisions
Restrained
Shy/timid
Talks to self
Worry

Essential Nutrients to Strengthen the Spleen Meridian

Vitamin A, vitamin C, calcium, chromium, protein, berries, asparagas, biofla-
vonoids, rutin, hesparin, hawthorn berries, oranges, root vegetables, and sugar.

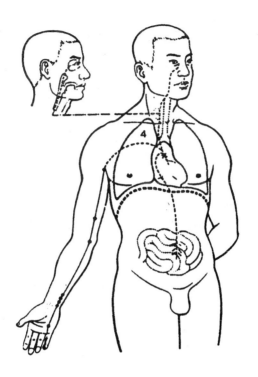

FIGURE 4-5

THE HEART MERIDIAN (HT)

THE HEART MERIDIAN (HT)

Energy disturbance in the heart meridian affecting the Physical and pysiological level can cause the following:

Angina-like pains
Chest pains
Discomfort when reclining
Dizziness
Dry throat
Excessive perspiration
Feverishness
Headache
Heart palpitation
Insomnia—unable to fall asleep
When awakened in the middle
    of sleep

Heaviness in the chest
Hot palms and soles
Irritability
Mental disorders
Nervousness
Pain along the left arm
Pain along the scapula
Pain and fullness in the chest
Pain in the eye
Poor circulation
Shortness of breath
Shoulder pains

Energy disturbance in the heart meridian affecting the cellular level can cause the following:

Abusive nature
Aggression
Anger
Bad manners
Compassion and love
Compulsive behaviors
Does not like to make friends
Does not trust anyone
Easily upset
Excessive laughing or crying

Guilt
Hostility
Insecurity
Joy
Lack of emotions
overexcitement
Lack of love and compassion
Sadness
Self-confidence
Type A personality

Essential Nutrients to Strengthen the Heart Meridian

Calcium, vitamin C, vitamin E, fatty acids, selenium, potassium, sodium, iron, and B complex.

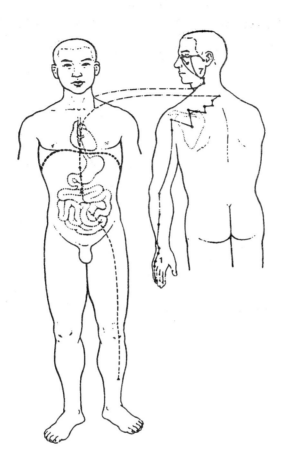

FIGURE 4-6

THE SMALL INTESTINE MERIDIAN (SI)

THE SMALL INTESTINE MERIDIAN (SI)

Energy disturbance in the small intestine meridian affecting physical and physiological levels can give rise to the following symptoms:

Abdominal fullness
Abdominal pain
Acne on the upper back
Bad breath
Bitter taste in the mouth
Constipation
Diarrhea
Distention of lower abdomen
Dry stool
Frozen shoulder
Knee pain
Night sweats

Numbness of the back of the shoulder and arm
Numbness of the mouth and tongue
Pain along the lateral aspect of the shoulder and arm
Pain in the neck
Pain radiating around the waist
Shoulder pain
Sore throat
Stiff neck

Energy disturbance in the small intestine meridian affecting the cellular level can cause the following:

Insecurity
Absentmindedness
Becoming too involved with details
Day dreaming
Easily annoyed
Emotional instability
Feeling of abandonment
Feeling shy
Having a tendency to be introverted and easily hurt
Irritability

Excessive joy or lack of joy
Lacking- confidence
Over excitement
Paranoia
Poor concentration
Sadness
Sighing
Sorrow
Suppressing deep sorrow

Essential Nutrients to Strengthen the Small Intestine Meridian

Vitamin B complex, vitamin D, vitamin E, acidophilus, yoghurt, fibers, fatty acids, wheat germ and whole grains.

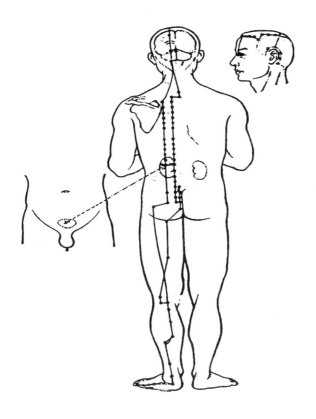

FIGURE 4-7
URINARY BLADDER MERIDIAN (UB)

URINARY BLADDER MERIDIAN (UB)

Energy disturbance in the Urinary Bladder meridian affecting physical and physiological levels can give rise to the following symptoms:

Arthritis of little finger & toe
Bloody urine
Burning or painful urination
Chills and fever
Disease of the eye
Frequent urination
Headaches at the back of the neck
Loss of bladder control
Lower backache and stiffness
lower abdominal discomfort
Mental disorders
Muscle wasting
Nasal congestion
Pain in the inner canthus
Pain and/or spasms along back
    of the leg, foot and lateral
        part of the sole & toes
Pain in the ankle (lateral part)
Pain along the meridian
Retention of urine
Sciatic neuralgia
Spasm behind the knee
Spasms of the calf muscles
Stiff neck
Weakness in the rectum and
    rectal muscle

Energy disturbance in the bladder meridian affecting the cellular level can cause the following:

Fright
Sadness
Disturbing and impure
   thoughts
Annoyed
Fearful
Unhappy
Frustrated
Highly irritable
Impatient
Inefficient
Insecure
Reluctant
Restless

Essential Nutrients to Strengthen the Bladder Meridian

Vitamin C, A, E, B complex, especially B_1, calcium, amino acids and trace minerals.

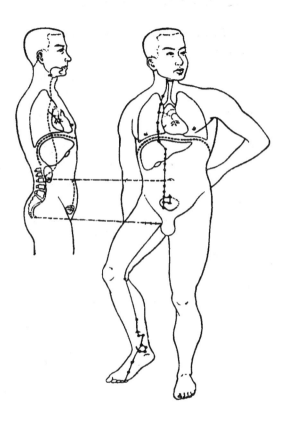

FIGURE   4-8

THE KIDNEY MERIDIAN (KI)

THE KIDNEY MERIDIAN (KI)

Energy disturbance in the kidney meridian affecting physical and physiological levels can give rise to the following symptoms:

Bags under the eyes
Blurred vision
Burning or painful urination
Chronic diarrhea
Coldness in the back
Cold feet
Crave salt
Dark circles under the eyes
Dryness of the mouth
Excessive sleeping
Excessive salivation
Excessive thirst
Facial edema
Fatigue
Fever with chills
Frequent urination
Impotence
Irritability
Light- headedness
Lower backache

Motor impairment
Muscular atrophy of the
   foot
Nagging mild asthma
Nausea
Pain in the sole of the foot
Pain in the posterior aspect
   of the leg or thigh
Pain in the ears
Poor memory
Poor concentration
Poor appetite
Puffy eyes
Ringing in the ears
Sore throat
Spasms of the ankle and
   feet
Swelling in the legs
Swollen ankles and vertigo

Energy disturbance in the kidney meridian affecting the cellular level can cause the following:

Fear
Terror
Caution
Confused

Indecision
Paranoia
Seeks attention
Unable to express feelings

Essential Nutrients to Strengthen the Kidney Meridian

Vitamins A, E, B, essential fatty acids, amino acids, sodium chloride (table salt), trace minerals, calcium and iron.

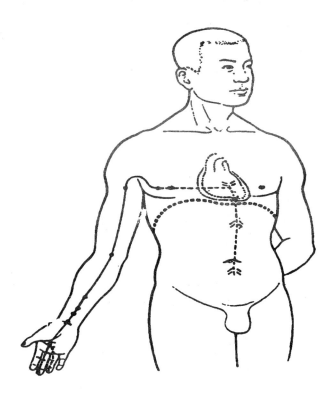

FIGURE 4-9

THE PERICARDIUM MERIDIAN (PC)

THE PERICARDIUM MERIDIAN (PC)

Energy disturbance in the pericardium meridian affecting physical and physiological levels can give rise to the following symptoms:

Chest pain
Contracture of the arm or elbow
Excessive appetite
Fainting spells
Flushed face
Frozen shoulder
Fullness in the chest
Heaviness in the chest
Hot palms and soles
Impaired speech
Irritability
Motor impairment of the tongue
Nausea

Nervousness
Pain in the anterior part of the thigh
Pain in the eyes
Pain in the medial part of the knee
Palpitation
Restricting movements
Sensation of hot or cold
Slurred speech
Spasms of the elbow and arm

Energy Disturbance in the Pericardium Meridian Affecting the Cellular Level Can Cause the Following:

Extreme joy
Fear of heights
Heaviness in the chest due to emotional overload
Heaviness in the head
Hurt
Imbalance in sexual energy like never having enough sex
In some cases no desire for sex

Jealousy
Light sleep with dreams
Manic disorders
Over- excitement
Regret
Sexual tension
Shock
Stubbornness
Various phobias

Essential Nutrients to Strengthen the Pericardium Meridian

Vitamin E, Vitamin C, Chromium, Manganese, Lotus seed, and Trace Minerals.

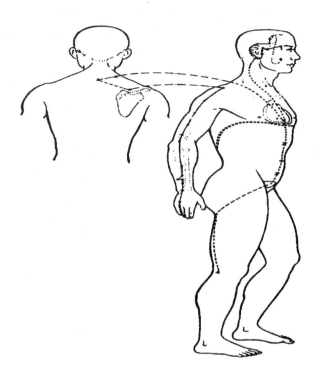

FIGURE 4-10

THE TRIPLE WARMER MERIDIAN (TW)

THE TRIPLE WARMER MERIDIAN (TW)

Energy disturbance in the triple warmer meridian affecting physical and physiological levels can give rise to the following symptoms:

Abdominal pain
Always feels hungry even
   after eating a full meal
Constipation
Deafness
Distention
Dysuria
Edema
Enuresis
Excessive thirst
Excessive hunger
Fever in the late evening
Frequent urination
Indigestion

Hardness and fullness in
   the lower abdomen
Pain in the medial part of
   the knee
Pain in the shoulder and
   upper arm
Pain behind the ear
Pain in the cheek and jaw
Redness in the eye
Shoulder pain
Swelling and pain in the
   throat
Vertigo

Energy disturbance in the triple warmer meridian affecting the cellular level can cause the following:

Depression
Deprivation
Despair
Emptiness

Excessive Emotion
Grief
Hopelessness
Phobias

Essential nutrients to strengthen the triple warmer meridian

Iodine, trace minerals, vitamin C, calcium, fluoride, radish, onion, zinc, vanadium, and water.

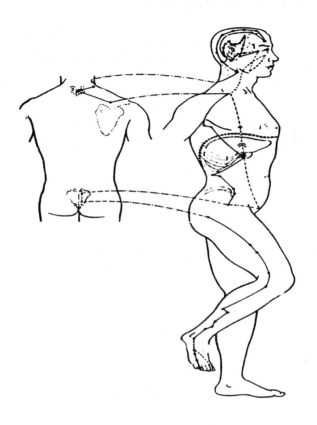

FIGURE   4-11

THE GALL BLADDER MERIDIAN (GB)

THE GALL BLADDER MERIDIAN (GB)

Energy disturbance in the gall bladder meridian affecting physical and physiological levels can give rise to the following symptoms:

A heavy sensation in the right
  upper part of the abdomen
Abdominal bloating
Alternating fever and chills
Ashen complexion
Bitter taste in the mouth
Burping after meals
Chills
Deafness
Dizziness
Fever
Headaches on the sides of the
  head
Heartburn after fatty foods
Hyperacidity
Moving arthritis
Pain in the jaw

Nausea with fried foods
Pain in the eye
Pain in the hip
Pain and cramps along the
  anterolateral wall
Poor digestion of fats
Sciatic neuralgia
Sighing
Stroke-like condition
Swelling in the submaxillary
  region
Tremors
Twitching
Vision disturbances
Vomiting
Yellowish complexion

Energy Disturbance in the Gall Bladder Meridian Affecting the Cellular Level
Can Cause the Following:

Aggression
Complaining all the time
Rage

Fearful, finding faults with
  others
Unhappiness.

Essential Nutrients to Strengthen the Gall Bladder Meridian

Vitamin A, apples, lemon, calcium, linoleic acids and oleic acids (for
example, pine nuts, olive oil).

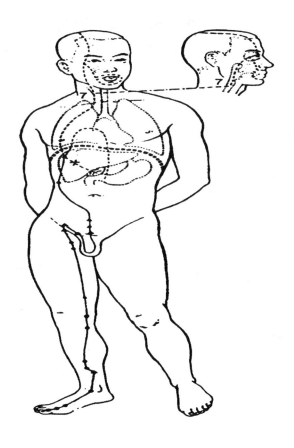

FIGURE 4-12

THE LIVER MERIDIAN (LIV)

THE LIVER MERIDIAN (LIV)

Energy disturbance in the liver meridian affecting physical and physiological levels can give rise to the following symptoms:

Abdominal pain
Blurred vision
Chemical sensitivities
Dark urine
Dizziness
Enuresis
Bright colored bleeding during
    menses
Feeling of obstruction in the
    throat
Fever
Hard lumps in the upper
    abdomen
Headache at the top of the head
Hernia
Hemiplegia
Irregular menses

Jaundice
Loose stools
Pain in the intercostal region
Pain in the breasts
Pain in the lower abdomen
Paraplegia
PMS
Reproductive organ
    disturbances
Retention of urine
Seizures
Spasms in the extremities
Stroke-like condition
Tinnitus
Vertigo
Vomiting.

Energy disturbance in the liver meridian affecting the cellular level can cause the following:

Anger
Irritability
Aggression
Assertion

Rage
Shouting
Talking loud
Type   A personality

Essential Nutrients to Strengthen the Liver Meridian

Beets, green vegetables, vitamin A, trace minerals, vitamin F

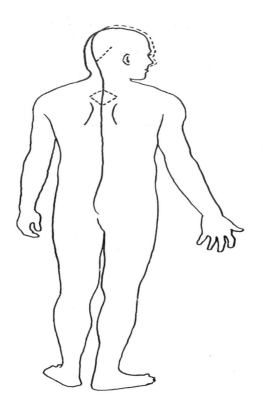

FIGURE 4-13

THE GOVERNING VESSEL MERIDIAN (GV)

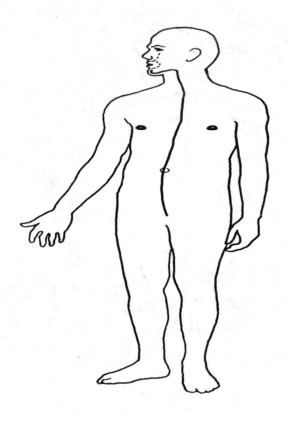

FIGURE 4-14

THE CONCEPTION VESSEL MERIDIAN (CV, REN)

THE GOVERNING VESSEL MERIDIAN (GV)

Energy disturbance in the governing vessel meridian affecting physical, physiological and psychological levels can give rise to various mixed symptoms of other yang meridians.

This channel supplies the brain and spinal region and intersects the liver channel at the vertex. Obstruction of its Chi may result in symptoms such as stiffness and pain along the spinal column. Deficient Chi in the channel may produce a heavy sensation in the head, vertigo and shaking. Energy blockages in this meridian (which passes through the brain) may be responsible for certain mental disorders. Febrile diseases are commonly associated with the governing vessel channel and because one branch of the channel ascends through the abdomen, when the channel is unbalanced, its Chi rushes upward toward the heart. Symptoms such as colic, constipation, enuresis, hemorrhoids and functional infertility may result.

THE CONCEPTION VESSEL MERIDIAN (CV, REN)

Energy disturbance in the conception vessel meridian affecting physical, physiological and psychological levels can give rise to various mixed symptoms of other yin meridians.

The conception vessel channel is the confluence of the Yin channels. Therefore, abnormality along the conception vessel channel will appear principally in pathological symptoms of the Yin channels, especially symptoms associated with the liver and kidneys. Its function is closely related with pregnancy and, therefore, has intimate links with the kidneys and uterus. If its Chi is deficient, infertility or other disorders of the urogenital system may result. Leukorrhea, irregular menstruation, colic, low libido, impotency, male and female infertility are associated with the conception vessel channel.

Any allergen can cause blockage in one or more meridians at the same time. If it is causing blockages in only one meridian, the patient may demonstrate symptoms related to that particular meridian. The intensity of the symptoms will depend on the severity of the blockage. The patient may suffer from one symptom, many symptoms or all the symptoms of this blocked meridian.

Sometimes a patient can have many meridians blocked at the same time. In such cases, the patient may demonstrate a variety of symptoms, one symptom from each meridian or many symptoms from certain meridians and one or two from other. Some patients with blockage in one meridian can demonstrate just one symptom from the list, but it may be with great intensity.

Some patients, even though they have energy disturbances in multiple meridians, may not show any symptoms. Such patients might have a better immune system than others. Variations with all these possibilities can make diagnosis difficult in some cases.

5

NAET® TESTING PROCEDURES

W hen a person comes close to the energy field of a substance, if that energy field happens to be incompatible to the individual, then a repulsion of the two energy fields take place. The substance that is capable of producing the repulsion between the energy fields of the individual and the substance itself is considered an allergen to the particular individual. We frequently go near allergens and interact with their energies without recognizing this repulsive action, whether from foods, drinks, chemicals, environmental substances, animals or other humans. This causes energy disturbances in the meridians; thereby causing imbalances in the body. The imbalances cause illnesses, which create disorganization in body functions. The disorganization of the body and its functions involve the vital organs, their associated muscle groups, and nerve roots which can give rise to brain disorders. To prevent the allergen from causing further disarray after producing the initial blockage, the brain sends messages to every cell of the body to reject the presence of the allergen. This rejection will appear as repulsion, and the repulsion will produce different symptoms related to the affected organs.

Our body has an amazing way of telling us when we are in trouble. If we went for help at the earliest hint of need, we would save ourselves from unnecessary pain and agony. As a matter of habit, we often have to be hurting severely before we seek help. This applies to chemical allergies, too. If we have a way to identify the allergens that can possibly cause reactions on our body way before we get exposed to them, we can simply avoid them and won't have to suffer the consequences. Now we have a way to do just that through NAET® testing procedures (NAET® Testing procedures are described in the following pages).

When we go near allergens, we may receive various clues from the brain if we are very aware of our own body sensitivities. Some of the examples of such body awareness are: itching, sneezing, coughing spells, stretching the body, yawning, feeling of fatigue, pain anywhere in the body, etc. These can happen when we come near an allergen. We can demonstrate these changes by testing the strength of any part of the body in the presence and absence of the allergen. A strong muscle of the arm, hand or leg can be used for this test. Test a strong muscle for its strength away from the allergen, and then test it again in the presence of the allergen and compare the strength. The muscle will stay strong without any allergen near the body, but will weaken in the presence of an allergen. This response of the muscle can be used to our advantage to demonstrate the presence of an allergen near us.

NEUROMUSCULAR SENSITIVITY TESTING
(NST-NAET®)

NST is one of the tools used by NAET® specialists to test imbalances and allergies in the body. The same muscle response testing can also be used to detect various allergens that cause imbalances in the body.

Neuromuscular sensitivity testing can be performed in the following ways (Illustrations of different types of NST can be seen on the following pages).

1. Standard NST can be done in standing, sitting or lying positions.

2. The "Oval Ring Test" can be used in testing yourself, and on a very strong person with a strong arm.

3. Surrogate testing can be used to test an infant, invalid person, extremely strong or very weak person, or an animal. The surrogate's muscle is tested by the tester, and the subject maintains skin-to-skin contact with the surrogate while being tested. The surrogate does not get affected by the testing. NAET® treatments can also be administered through the surrogate very effectively without causing any interference with the surrogate's energy.

NST PROCEDURE

Two people are required to perform standard neuromuscular sensitivity testing: the tester, and the subject. The subject can be tested lying down, standing, or sitting. The lying-down position is

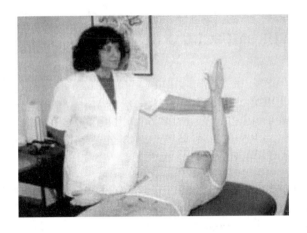

**FIGURE 5-1
NST WITHOUT ALLERGEN**

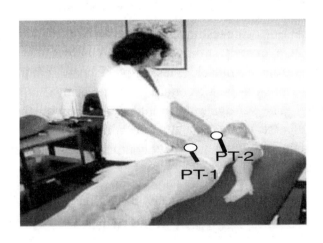

**FIGURE 5-2
INITIAL BALANCING**

the most convenient for both tester and subject; it also achieves more accurate results.

Step 1:   The subject lies on a firm surface with the left arm raised 45-90 degrees to the body with the palm facing outward and the thumb pointing toward the big toe.

Step 2: The tester stands on the subject's (right) side. The subject's right arm is kept to his/her side with the palm either kept open to the air, or in a loose fist. The fingers should not touch any material, fabric or any part of the table the arm is resting on because this can give wrong test results. The tester's left palm is contacting the subject's left wrist (Figure 5-1).

Step 3: It is essential to test a strong predetermined muscle (PDM) to get accurate results. The tester using the left arm tries to push the raised arm toward the subject's left big toe. The subject resists the push. The arm, or predetermined indicator muscle, remains strong if the subject is well balanced at the time of testing. If the muscle or raised arm is weak and gives way under pressure without the presence of an allergen, either the subject is not balanced, or the tester is performing the test improperly; for example, the tester might be trying to overpower the subject. The subject does not need to gather up strength from other muscles in the body to resist the tester. Only 5 to 10 pounds of pressure needs to be applied for three to five seconds. If the muscle shows weakness, the tester will be able to judge the difference with only that small amount of pressure.

Step 4: This step is used if the patient is found to be out of balance as indicated by the PDM presenting weak without the presence of an allergen. The tester then uses the balancing points by placing the fingertips of right hand at Point 1. The left hand is placed on Point 2 (see below and figure 5-2). The tester massages these two points gently clockwise with the fingertips about 20-30 seconds, and then repeats steps 2 and 3. If the PDM tests strong, continue on to step 5.

MORE ON STEP-4

Point 1:

Name of the point: Sea of Energy

Location: Two finger-breadths below the navel, on the midline. According to Oriental medical theory, this is where the energy of the body is stored in abundance. When the body senses any danger around its energy field or when the body experiences energy disturbances, the energy supply is cut short and stored here. If you massage clockwise on that energy reservoir point, the energy will come out of this storage and travel to the part of the body where it is needed.

Point 2:

Name of the point: Dominating Energy

Location: In the center of the chest on the midline of the body, level with the fourth intercostal space. This is the energy dispenser department. According to Oriental medical theory, when the energy rises from the Sea of Energy, it goes straight to the Dominating Energy point. This is the point that controls and regulates the energy circulation or Chi flow in the body. From this point, the energy is distributed to different meridians, organs, tissues and cells as needed to help remove the energy disturbances in those affected areas.

This is done by forcing energy circulation to flow from the energy distribution area (Point-2 on figure-2) to the affected meridian, then to the affected tissue in the meridian moving the energy into general circulation or we can say "move the energy from inside out". Continue this procedure for 30 seconds to one minute and repeat the NST. If the NST is found weak repeat the procedure until it gets strong. Check NST every 30 seconds. In a very sick individual it may be necessary to repeat this procedure for three or four times before the PDM becomes strong.

Step 5: If the PDM remains strong when tested - a sign that the subject is balanced - then the tester should put the suspected allergen into the palm of the subject's resting hand. When the subject's fingertips touch the allergen, the sensory receptors sense the allergen's charges and relay the message to the brain. If it is an incompatible charge, the strong PDM will go weak. If the charges are compatible to the body, the indicator muscle will remain strong. This way, you can test any number of items to determine the compatible and incompatible charges.

Much practice is needed to test and sense the differences properly. If you can't test properly or effectively the first few times, don't get discouraged. Practice makes one perfect.

NST is one of the most reliable methods of allergy tests, and it is fairly easy to learn and practice in every day life. The tester will develop confidence after getting enough practice. It also cuts out expensive laboratory work.

After considerable practice, some people are able to test very efficiently using these methods. It is very important for the chemically sensitive people to learn this simple testing technique to screen out the allergies before he/she gets exposed to them in order to prevent unexpected allergic reactions. After receiving

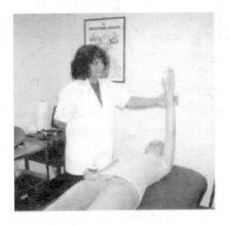

**FIGURE 5-3
NST WITH ALLERGEN**

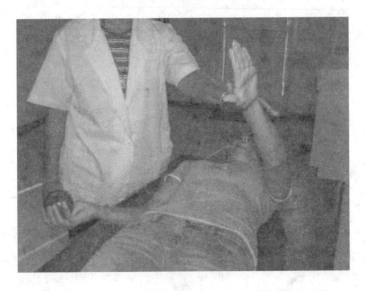

**FIGURE 5-4
NST WEAK WITH ALLERGEN**

NAET® Basic treatments from a trained NAET® practitioner, you can begin to test and screen your daily encountering allergens before using them. Then the offending substances can easily be avoided, or if it is unavoidable, be treated. Hundreds of new allergens are thrown into the world daily by chemical manufacturers who do not understand the predicament of allergic people. If you want to live in this world looking and feeling normal, you have to learn self-testing. It is not practical for anyone to treat thousands of allergens from their surroundings or go to an NAET® practitioner every day for the rest of one's life. If you learn to detect the allergies on your own, after treating for NAET® basics you can easily avoid most other allergens by testing prior to exposures.

"OVAL RING TEST" OR "O RING TEST"

The "Oval Ring Test" or "O Ring Test" can be used in self-testing. This can also be used to test a subject, if the subject is very strong physically with a strong arm and the tester is a physically weak person. (See figure 5-7)

Step 1: The tester makes an "O" shape by opposing the little finger and thumb on the same hand (finger pad to finger pad). Then, with the index finger of the other hand he/she tries to separate the "O" ring against pressure. If the ring separates easily, the tester needs to be balanced as described above.

Step 2: If the "O" ring remains inseparable and strong, hold an allergen in the other hand, by the fingertips, and perform step 1 again. If the "O" ring separates easily, the person is allergic to the substance in the hand. If the "O" ring remains strong, the substance is not an allergen.

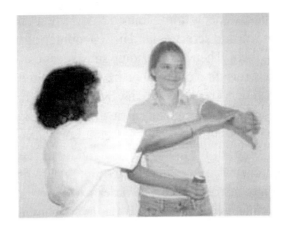

FIGURE 5-5
NST IN STANDING POSITION

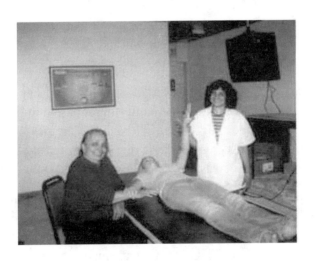

FIGURE 5-6
TESTING THROUGH A SURROGATE

Chapter 5

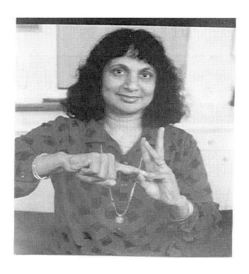

FIGURE 5-7
"O" RING TESTING

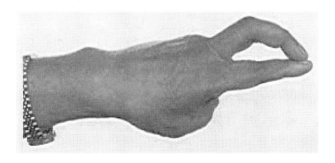

FIGURE 5- 8
FINGER ON FINGER TESTING

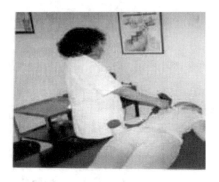

FIGURE 5-10
NAET TREATMENT

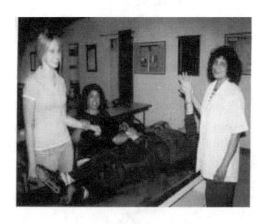

FIGURE 5-11
EXTENDED SURROGATE TESTING

After considerable practice, some people are able to test very efficiently using these methods. It is very important for allergic people to learn some form of self-testing technique to screen out contact with possible allergens to prevent allergic reactions in order to have freedom to live in this chemically polluted world. After receiving the basic 30-40 treatments from a NAET® practitioner, a person can test and avoid unexpected allergens. Hundreds of new allergens are thrown into the world daily by people who do not understand the predicament of allergic people. If you want to live in this world looking and feeling normal among normal people, you need to learn how to test on your own. It is not practical for people to treat thousands of allergens from their surroundings or go to a NAET® practitioner every day. If you learn to detect your allergies on your own after treating for NAET® basics, you can live without many health problems.

A TIP TO MASTER SELF-TESTING

Find two items, one that you are allergic to and another that you are not, for example an apple and a banana.

You are allergic to the apple and not allergic to the banana. Hold the apple in the right hand and do the "Oval Ring Test" as shown in the figure 5-7. The ring easily breaks. The first few times if it didn't break, make it happen intentionally. Now hold the banana and do the same test. This time the ring doesn't break. Put the banana down; rub your hands together for 30 seconds. Take the apple and repeat the testing. Practice this until you can sense the difference. When you can feel the difference between these two items you can test anything around you.

SURROGATE TESTING

This method can be very useful to test and determine the allergies of an infant, a child, a hyperactive child, an autistic child, disabled person, an unconscious person, an extremely strong, and a very weak person. You can also use this method to test an animal, plant, and a tree.

TESTING THROUGH AN EXTENDED SURROGATE

Extended surrogate testing is used when the patient is uncooperative, i.e. hyperactive, autistic, or frightened. Three people are needed for this test as shown in Figure 5-11. NAET® treatments can be administered through the extended surrogate very effectively without causing any interference to the surrogate's energy.

The surrogate's muscle is tested by the tester. It is very important to remember to maintain skin-to-skin contact between the surrogate and the subject during the procedure. If you do not, then the surrogate will receive the results of testing and treatment.

The testing or treatment does not affect the surrogate as long as the subject maintains uninterrupted skin-to-skin contact with the surrogate.

NST can be used to test any substance for allergies. Even human beings can be tested for each other in this manner. When allergic to another human (father, mother, son, daughter, grandfather, grandmother, spouse, caretaker, baby sitter, etc.) you or your child could experience similar symptoms just as you would with foods, chemicals, or materials.

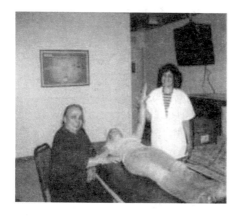

FIGURE 5-12
PERSON TO PERSON TESTING (A TO B)

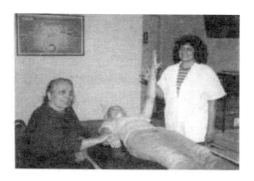

FIGURE 5-13
PERSON TO PERSON TESTING (B TO A)

ABOUT PERSON-TO-PERSON ALLERGIES

If people are allergic to each other, the allergy can affect a person in various ways: If the father and/or mother is allergic to the child, or child allergic to a parent or parents, the child can get sick or remain sick indefinitely. The same things can happen to the parents. If the husband is allergic to the wife or wife towards the husband, they might fight all the time and/or their health can be affected. The same things can happen among other family members. It is important to test family members and other immediate associates with your child for possible allergy, and if found, they should be treated for each other.

TESTING PERSON-TO-PERSON ALLERGIES

The subject lies down and touches the other person he or she wants tested (Figures 5-12 and 5-13). The tester pushes the arm of the subject in steps 2 and 3 above. If the subject is allergic to the second person, the indicator muscle goes weak. If the subject is not allergic, the indicator muscle remains strong. This is done through a surrogate in autistic children. Sometimes, one needs to test an autistic or hyperactive child through an extended surrogate because the child may be violent or too strong for one surrogate to handle.

QUESTION RESPONSE TESTING (QRT)

The brain and nervous system work around the clock to take care of the body's needs, watching and protecting it from any physical, physiological and/or emotional harm. The electromagnetically sensitive nervous system is very efficient in communicating with each nerve cell in the body in complete coordination, and also has the ability to connect and communicate with the electromagnetic forces of other living or nonliving beings of the universe from any distance. So, we can trust our brain to find the best answers to our questions about our health.

In other words, we can ask our brain any question and it will give us the correct answer related to our health. Each cell in our brain and the nervous system is built uniquely with specialized cell materials which have the ability to measure and assess the energy differences of various things from our internal or external environments: disturbed body functions, substances from our environment causing energy blockages, emotional disturbances, good and bad thoughts, vibrations, temperature change that disturbs our energy flow or circulation in the body, etc. We can test the subject by asking these specific questions. This can be also done through a surrogate. In such case the patient and the surrogate should maintain skin-to-skin contact with each other during testing.

NAET®-QRT PROCEDURE

Since we are asking the subconscious to help us find the answer to our questions, the tester should ask the questions silently in his/her mind in order to prevent the conscious mind from confusing the subconscious from giving the right answer. We can use the same PDM we used earlier as a source of reference points to verify our answers that we receive from the brain. Subconscious and conscious minds are part of the brain. Conscious mind thinks, feels, gets tired, gets sleepy, etc. whereas, the subconscious mind never thinks, gets tired or sleeps. It gathers information about everything regarding the person and stores the information in the memory bank. So the subconscious mind knows everything that has happened to the person from day one of his/her life until the present. Subconscious mind records every bit of knowledge that is collected during the life of the person and stores it safely to recall in the future if it ever became necessary. We are going to use information from this storage to help improve our health.

ASKING QUESTIONS

The tester will ask questions about your health in his/her mind silently while testing your PDM for its weakening or strengthening effect.

This time, we are replacing the food or allergenic substance with the question(s). So the question is the sample. We should make a list of questions that we need to ask about your health before we begin performing NST. The question should be asked about the health history, childhood history, possible cause for the present health problem, the best treatment approach, etc. The brain cannot talk to us in words or sentences. We must create ways to extract answers from the brain. Then only we can communicate with the brain.

Ask a question silently then check the PDM for its strengthening or weakening effect. If the PDM is weak, the answer is interpreted as "yes."

If the PDM tests strong, the answer is a "no."

THE TECHNIQUES OF ASKING QUESTIONS

Let us look at some examples of questions to use while performing QRT. The examples might help you understand better. Let us say Ron is very sick for the past two weeks. He was coughing, wheezing, and fatigued.

Have Ron in the NST position without sample. Refer to figure-5-1. Here, the right hand is raised for testing and the left hand is kept open to the air or make a loose fist. The tester is asking pre-formulated questions silently in his/her mind about Ron's health. When the PDM shows a weak response, it will be taken as a "Yes"; when the PDM response is strong the interpretation is a "No".

Question: Is your present health problem triggered by an allergy? At the end of the question, perform NST on the PDM.

If the PDM goes weak, Ron's subconscious part of the brain is saying, "Yes, my present health problem is triggered by an allergy."

If the PDM remains strong, then the brain is saying, "No, my present health problem is not triggered by an allergy."

Lets say the PDM went weak in this case. So we shall continue with the questions:

Question: If your problem is triggered by an allergy, is that allergen a solid food?

Answer: Strong PDM indicates, "No, my problem is not triggered by a solid food."

Question: "Is your problem triggered by a liquid that you drink?"

Answer: Weak NST indicates a "Yes, It is a liquid"

Question: "If it is caused by drinking a liquid, do you drink this liquid daily?"

Answer: Weak NST indicates, "Yes, I drink this liquid daily"

Question: "If you drink this liquid daily, is it milk?"

Answer: Strong NST indicates, "No, it is not milk."

Question: "If you drink this liquid daily, is it fruit juice?"

Answer: Strong NST indicates, "No, it is not fruit juice."

Question: "If you drink this liquid daily, is it soup?"

Answer: Strong NST indicates, "No, it is not soup."

Question: "If you drink this liquid daily, is it any liquid medication?"

Answer: Strong NST indicates, "No, it is not liquid medication."

Question: "If you drink this liquid daily, is it bottled water?"

Answer: Strong NST indicates, "No, it is not bottled water."

Question: "If you drink this liquid daily, is it the city water or tap water?"

Answer: Weak NST indicates, "Yes, it is the city water (tap water.)"

Question: "Is the drinking of tap water causing your cough?"

Answer: Weak NST indicates, "Yes, it is causing my cough."

Question: "Is the drinking of tap water causing your wheezing?"

Answer: Weak NST indicates, "Yes, it is causing my wheezing."

Question: "Is the drinking of tap water causing your fatigue?"

Answer: Weak NST indicates, "Yes, it is causing my fatigue."

Get a sample of the tap water and perform NAET® on Ron for the tap water.

When he clears the allergy for the tap water, his symptoms will reduce or disappear.

Using this method the tester can screen each and every food, drink, vitamins, medications, fabrics, chemicals, etc. before the chemically sensitive person exposes herself or himself to the substance. If you find them as allergens, test more items until you can find non-allergic products. Of course, you have the option to treat for them and make non-allergic or avoid them and never use them again.

If we can teach these simple testing skills to all chemically sensitive people, their families, their guardians, their caretakers, and their Doctors, as well as encourage them to use non-allergic products or NAET® treated products in their daily use, chemically sensitive person can also lead a healthy and happy life.

As mentioned earlier, muscle response testing is one of the tools used by kinesiologists. Practiced in this country since 1964, it was originated by Dr. George Goodheart and his associates. The late Dr. John F. Thie advocated this method through the "Touch for Health" Foundation in Malibu, California. For more information and books available on the subject; interested readers can write to "Touch For Health" Foundation.

Freedom From Chemical Sensitivities

6

NAET® Home-Help

Y ou have seen how allergies can interfere with the lives, how allergies can complicate your existence and take the pleasure out of living. You will be amazed to find that many of the medical problems you suffer may have allergies as their origins. Using the methods described in Chapter 5, you can learn to test your allergies and discover the causes of most of your common illnesses or so called "incurable" disorders.

If you learn the testing procedures and practice at home, it won't be long before you find out that most of your health problems (or your loved one's) have their roots in your daily diets, or clothes, even in the vitamins you were using which you thought were helping you to live healthy and well.

How surprised will you be when you discover (for example) that:

Your 20-year-old eczema was due to an allergy to eggs and aggravated by eating eggs and chicken products or due to dried beans (proteins) taken to supplement your diet with enough protein?

An allergy to your soft, expensive feather pillow was causing your chronic sinusitis and neck pains.

Your constant lower backache was due to an allergy to the pesticide that was sprayed regularly once a week in your house for years to keep the ants and roaches away.

Your daily, nagging morning headaches were due to an allergy to the smell from the coffee your husband brewed in the morning before you woke up and brought you a cup so lovingly to the bed routinely.

Your joint pains and arthritis were due to an allergy to the food bleach that you consumed on a daily basis via bleached white flour, white rice and white breads at most meals.

The fatigue you experienced every morning was contributed by an allergy to the diet chocolate pudding you ate at bedtime to keep your weight off and to maintain a good figure.

Your on-going personality disorder, behavior disorder, attention-deficit disorder, anger, frustration, depression and mood swings were due to an allergy to the beef jerky you snacked on frequently during the small breaks you took between your computer work thinking that the computer radiation was the cause of the above problems.

The rough, scaly skin was actually due to an allergy to the shrimp cocktail you enjoyed at least four times a week at the "happy hour" time at the hotel you worked as a refreshment manager at the VIP lounge.

Your unresolved bad breath, low energy and brain fog that developed seven years ago after an extensive dental work were contributed by an allergy to mercury that was used in the dental filling composite put in the mouth.

Your abdominal bloating around your menstrual cycle was due to an allergy to the tampons and sanitary napkins you used.

Your child's chronic bronchitis was probably due to an allergy to that one glass of milk he drank every morning, and when he was found to be allergic to chlorox and after the elimination of an allergy to chlorox his chronic bronchitis cleared up nicely.

Your child's hyperactivity and poor attention span were caused by an allergy to the coloring pencils and crayons he uses to color in the school every day.

Your child's Dr. Jekyll and Mr. Hyde-like behavior was caused by an allergy to the fabric softener you used with every wash to reduce the static electricity from the washed clothes.

Your child's frequent colds and sore throat were due to an allergy to the city water he drinks in school.

Your husband's two-month-old walking pneumonia was due to an allergy to the yoghurt he eats daily for lunch at work.

Your irritating yeast-like infection was due to the allergy to the toilet paper you use daily.

Children are more susceptible to get chronic diseases due to chemical toxicity. Evidence is increasing that toxic chemicals in the environment contribute to causation of disease in children. Many studies have been done in this area to prove it. People are surrounded by a large and ever increasing number of chemicals.

Children get affected more than the adults for various reasons. Many of the chemicals to which children are at risk of exposure have not been tested for their possible developmental toxicity. A report from EPA pointed out that there are 80,000 + chemicals are in commerce; 2,863 produced or imported in quantities of 1 million pounds or more per year (high production volume [HPV] chemicals); No basic toxicity information is publicly available for about half of HPV chemicals and Information on developmental toxicity is publicly available for fewer than 20% of HPV chemicals (EPA: Chemical Hazard Data Availability Study, 1998).

National Academy of Sciences reported that children are more heavily exposed and more vulnerable to many environmental chemicals than adults because of greater exposure proportionate to body mass–7 times more water per Kg per day; increased hand-to mouth activity; diminished ability to detoxify many chemicals naturally; heightened biological vulnerability–thalidomide, DES, fetal alcohol syndrome and more years of future life. (National Academy of Sciences, 1993).

Some researchers have found the causes of birth defects, asthma, learning disabilities, attention deficit hyperactive disorders, autism and a few genetic disorders due to following reasons: known indoor triggers include house dust, secondhand tobacco smoke, mold and mildew, cockroach droppings, certain pesticides, ambient air pollution–ozone and particulates and poor living conditions. Evidence for environmental causation of childhood cancer is noted due to radiation, solvents, especially benzene, parental employment in industries that use solvents–painting and printing, and pesticide exposure, especially prenatally.

Certain male reproductive disorders are suspected to have been happening from exposures to environmental hazards. Some of these disorders are: Low sperm counts, rising testicular cancer and increasing hypospadias. Some of the chemicals may be disrupting the hormonal and endocrine system. Definite answers and evidences have not been found to support the claim.

Certain neurodevelopmental disorders in adults and children are observed happening from exposures to environmental toxins such as lead, methyl mercury, polychlorinated biphenyls (PCBs), polybrominated biphenyls (PBBs), pesticides, insecticides, weed killer chemicals, etc. Early exposure to neurotoxins may increase the risk of degenerative disease in later life such as Alzheimer's disease or Parkinson's disease. Neurodevelopmental disability is not limited to severe debilitating health conditions alone but it can include a vast number of mild to moderate health disorders which probably most people may not even relate or suspect to chemical toxicity. They may call these symptoms as "Something out of sorts" or "Something is not right" kind of feeling as in subclinical toxicity and symptoms. Often subclinical neurotoxicity can affect the health, well-being, intelligence and even the security of an entire population.

Dioxin is a known carcinogen and can cause cancer, especially breast cancer in sensitive people. When certain plastic containers or bottles heated in the microwave oven dioxin may be released from the plastics into the contents. Saran wrap is used by many people all over the world to cover the dish while cooking in the microwave. Some studies have shown saran wrap can release large amount of dioxin causing various health hazards. Some researchers advise us against using microwave ovens for cooking or heating foods. They believe the nutrition is altered in the foods cooked in the microwave oven. Today we live in a unusually fast paced society where time is very short for everyone even to run the most important daily chores. Since people do get hungry, they look for easy foods like TV dinners, cup of noodles and microwavable pizza and things like that. To heat up the foods the microwave ovens become a necessity or such people or the choice is to eat cold TV dinners. When the food is heated up in the microwave oven, whether they get nutrition or not, food tastes good and they could save a lot of time to finish up other chores. So, the life of 21st century has become very different from our ancestors where the house-wives spent entire day from dawn to dusk preparing food for the family. But the life has changed now. It is not practical for someone to stay home and cook whole day because husband and wife, both have to work outside home to meet the growing expenses. So it is not practical for many people to give up using microwave ovens even if they cost them their health. The next best thing will be to use the right way of heating foods. Glasswares, corning wares are suggested in microwave cooking rather than other utensils. If plastic containers are used it is advisable not to cover them with plastic sheets or saran wap.

The other day I watched an interesting program on TV. Dr. Edward Fujimoto from Castle hospital was on a TV program explaining this health hazard we are facing about dioxin poisoning. (He is the manager of the Wellness Program at Mary Hitchcock Hospital in Hanover, NH.). He was talking how bad they are for us. He said that we should not be heating our food in the microwave oven using plastic containers at all. This applies to foods that contain fat mainly. He said that the combination of fat, high heat and plastics releases dioxin into the food and ultimately into the cells of our bodies leading to dioxin poisoning. Instead, he recommends using glass, or ceramic containers for heating food. We get the same results...without dioxin. TV dinners, instant soups, etc, should be taken out of their original containers and heated in the less hazardous containers made from above materials. As soon as I heard his talk the first thing I did was treat the dioxin and combination with heat, cold, and plastics immediately using NAET®. Even though I do not use much of microwave cooking, when we eat out we would never know how the restaurant is preparing or heating our food before it comes to our plate.

Paper containers or wrappers are OK to use in the microwave provided we know what is in the paper. Recycling of old papers is encouraged by all cities lately. When the paper goods and newspapers are recycled, the chemical contents are also recycled causing chemically sensitive people to get sicker than before upon using the recycled goods. Several of my patients suffered from asthma, headaches, migraines, arthritis, general fatigue, indigestion, gastric reflux disorders, etc. upon handling recycled paper products. It took a lot of detective work to trace their problems to recycled paper products. These recycled paper goods are encountered by us as in letters from government offices, schools and universities, utility bills (seen as gas, water, garbage and electric bills) and envelops, tour guide books and pamphlets, etc. After NAET® treatments for these products my patients did not suffer anymore short-term sicknesses. We are observing these patients closely for any long-term problems. So far we have not seen any long term hazards after the completion of NAET® on the said items. They continue to use the products without triggering any more previous problems. So probably dioxin poisoning could be prevented if the sensitive person get desensitized using NAET®. More research is needed in this area to understand the outcome..

Ninety percent human health disorders have some form of allergy involvement. Avoiding a substance is like running away from problem. That is not going to help you if you have to live in this world. If you did not treat with NAET® (I do not know any other form of treatment to permanently eliminate the adverse reaction of the substance from a body), these allergies can make you sick or at least put you "under the weather." If you learn how to test and find your allergies, if you can learn how to find the cause of your illnesses before these allergies cripple you, you could avoid a lot of mental agony. Now you have a way to do just that. You can test and detect your allergies within the privacy of your own home, using NAET® testing procedures. (Caution: If you are suffering from a major sickness, please see your doctor or appropriate specialist immediately and get evaluated first). Just by avoiding the allergens from your life, you will be able to live peacefully. If you must use the products, please see a practitioner who is trained in NAET®. If you take time to read this book, you will understand how to help yourself with mild to moderate allergies, because some self-help tips are given in this chapter. If you are one with many allergies, with severe symptoms, please consult an NAET® specialist right away to get a few NAET® treatments before you try self-help procedures. For complicated problems, you need to consult an appropriate specialist.

Everyone should be tested and treated for all NAET® Basic allergen groups, these are the very basic treatments. NAET® basic treatments include the basic essentials for life, the most commonly used food and enzymes from everyday life. If one is allergic to all the essential nutrients, he/she can become reactive to everything else around him/her. By eliminating the allergies to the essential nutrients, one's immunity will improve or maintain at a very high level, with the result, one may not get other allergies or allergy based illnesses as often as others who have not had the NAET® Basic treatments.

The purpose of this book is not to train a lay person in medical procedures. The real purpose of this book is to inform people about NAET® allergy elimination treatment, so that the chemically sensitive people can learn about the availability of such a treatment and, if interested, can locate the appropriate NAET® practitioner with proper NAET® training to help eliminate their allergies.

Information regarding a few important acupressure points, and NAET® energy balancing points are described in the following pages. These points and techniques, when used properly according to the accompanying instructions, might help to reduce or control your presenting acute and chronic allergic symptoms. If used properly, these points can be helpful in emergency situations.

A few home-help energy balancing applications are also discussed in this chapter, with illustrations. These balancing techniques are safe to use on people at any age and in any condition. When one maintains energy in a balanced state, the body may not experience any illness or adverse reactions. Just by balancing the body regularly, by maintaining a balanced state, many people have reported that they were able to keep their allergic reactions under control. Some have reported reduction in their allergy-related other health conditions as well.

But again I would like to make the reader aware that these are only energy balancing techniques and should not be confused with actual NAET® treatment procedures done with a trained NAET® specialist. These balancing techniques will not replace the need for a trained NAET® practitioner. These techniques alone are not sufficient to permanently eliminate your allergies. These procedures, when used properly as described in the following pages, will: help to improve overall health, reduce allergies and allergic reactions, help with allergy-related health problems, but will not eliminate your allergies permanently.

About NAET® Testing

In Chapter 5, you learned to test and find your allergies using NST and QRT. You have learned to test and identify allergens in general. If you want to be healthy, you are urged to practice these testing techniques and make a habit of testing everything you suspect before exposing yourself to them. When you identify the allergens, you may be able to avoid them easily.

I spent countless hours testing, determining, researching, and trying out all my NAET® discoveries on hundreds of people and pets before I began sharing them with others. I was a desperate patient myself sometime ago. I was told to learn to live with my chronic pains for the rest of my life. So I understand the pain of living with sickness and feeling trapped.

Now, we have a simple, safe, inexpensive, uncomplicated procedure to test allergies and allergy-related disorders with maximum accuracy.

You can test any type of allergen in this fashion. I am going to list a few commonly encountered, unsuspected, allergens below. When I tell someone to test each and every item before using, most people do not understand that one could be allergic to a vast number of everyday items around them. Most people, including some practitioners, miss unsuspected hidden allergens. These people continue to suffer from various health problems all along without a break.

NAET® Basic Allergens

1. BBF (Autonomic nervous system balance)
2. Egg mix (Proteins)
3. Calcium mix
4. Vitamin C mix
5. B complex
6. Sugar mix
7. Iron mix
8. Vitamin A mix
9. Minerals, water, drinking water, city water
10. Salt Mix
11. Grains
12. Yeast mix, yogurt and whey
13. Stomach acid
14. Digestive enzymes or Base
15. Hormones and other hormones

NAET Classic Allergens For Chemically Sensitive Person

The NAET Classic Allergens include the 15 NAET® Basic Allergens groups and 40 other major allergen groups. There are 55 major groups of allergens in the NAET classic allergens. The preferred order of treatments is given below. About 80 percent of one's allergic reactions towards substances will diminish if one clears 100 percent on all these allergens.

Hypothalamus

Chlorox

Chemical mix

Water

Organs

Food additive

Food colorings

Whiten-all

MSG

Alcohol

Artificial sweeteners

Coffee, chocolate and caffeine

Heavy metals

The items listed below are treated as needed and on a priority based protocol, which your NAET practitioner will explain to you.

Turkey

Neurotransmitters

Corn mix

Animal fat and body fat

Vegetable fat

Vitamin F

Spice mix 1 & 2

Dried Beans

Essential and nonessential amino acids

Startch mix

School / work material

Immunizations and vaccinations, or drugs

Fabrics

Plastics

Perfume

Check if any other smells bothering the person, if found treat them.

Molybdenum
Selenium
Cobalt
Baking powder/Baking soda
Nut mix-1 & nut mix-2

Fish and Shell fish

Whiten-all

Whey

Yogurt

Gelatin

Gum mix

Paper product

Fluoride

Vitamin E

Vitamin D

Vitamin K

Night shade vegetables

Pesticides

Insect bites/stings

Radiation

Inhalants

R.N.A. & D.N.A.

Tissues and secretions

Virus mix

Bacteria Mix

Parasites

Formaldehyde

Latex/plastics

Crude oil/Synthetic materials, etc.

Animal epithelial/dander/human hair

Smoking/nicotine

Dust/ dust mites

Allergy to people

Other chemicals not listed above

1. On the first visit: BBF (brain-body Balancing formula) - with this treatment there is nothing to avoid. Also treat the emotion for fear. Chemically sensitive people have fragile emotions. They suffer from various kinds of fears: fear of getting sick; fear of contacting chemicals in unexpected places; fear of meeting people (they may react to other's perfume, aftershave lotion, fabrics, fabric softener, detergent, body odor, smell of smoke or herbs or spices or garlic, etc. from other's clothes; fear of losing control due to chemical sensitivities); fear of not able to work; fear of not having enough money to live; fear of loneliness (Chemically sensitive people are afraid to live with people so they often live alone; fear of facing in the real world). You may use the list given at the back of this chapter to check the emotional blockages.

2.Egg Mix (egg white, egg yolk, chicken, and tetracycline).

You may only eat brown or white rice, pasta without eggs, vegetables, fruits, milk products, oils, beef, pork, fish, coffee, juice, soft drinks, water, and tea.

3. Milk and Calcium mix (breast milk, cow's milk, goat's milk, and calcium).

You may only eat cooked rice, cooked fruits and vegetables (like potato, squash, green beans, yams, cauliflower, sweet potato), chicken, red meat, and drink coffee, tea without milk, or calcium-free water.

4. Vitamin C mix (fruits, vegetables, vinegar, citrus, and berry).

You may only eat cooked white or brown rice, pasta without sauce, boiled or poached eggs, baked or broiled chicken, fish, red meat, brown toast, deep fried food, French fries, salt, oils, and drink coffee or water.

5. B complex vitamins (17 B-vitamins).

You may only eat cooked white rice, cauliflower raw or cooked, well cooked or deep fried fish, salt, white sugar, black coffee, French fries, and purified, non allergic water when treating for any of the B vitamins. Rice should be washed well before cooking. It should be cooked in lots of water and drained well to remove the fortified vitamins.

6. Sugar Mix (cane sugar, corn sugar, maple sugar, grape sugar, rice sugar, brown sugar, beet sugar, fructose, molasses, honey, dextrose, glucose, and maltose).

You may only eat white rice, pasta, vegetables, vegetable oils, meats, eggs, chicken, water, coffee, tea without milk.

7. Iron Mix (animal and vegetable sources, beef, pork, lamb, raisin, date, and broccoli).

You may only eat white rice without iron fortification, sour dough bread without iron, cauliflower, white potato, chicken light green vegetables (white cabbage, ice berg lettuce, white squash, yellow squash, and orange juice.

8. Vitamin A (animal and vegetable source, beta carotene, fish and shell fish).

You may eat only cooked rice, pasta, potato, cauliflower, red apples, chicken, water, and coffee.

9. Mineral Mix (magnesium, manganese, phosphorus, selenium, zinc, copper, cobalt, chromium, trace minerals, gold, germanium, vanadium, potassium, boron, and fluoride).

You may use only distilled water for washing, drinking, and showering. You may eat only cooked rice, vegetables, fruits, meats, eggs, milk, coffee, and tea. No root vegetables.

10. Salt Mix (sodium and sodium chloride, water filter water softener salts, and chemicals).

You may use distilled water for drinking and washing, cooked rice, fresh vegetables and fruits (except celery, carrots, beets, artichokes, romaine lettuce, and watermelon) meats, chicken, and sugars.

11. Grain Mix (wheat, gluten, corn, oats, millet, barley, and rice).

You may eat vegetables, fruits, meats, milk, and drink water. Avoid all products with gluten.

12. Yeast mix (brewer's yeast, and bakers yeast).

You may eat vegetables, meat, chicken, and fish. No fruits, no sugar products. Drink distilled water.

At this time start collecting a small portion of different food groups from every meal and self-balance your energy for the mixture of breakfast, lunch and dinner after each meal. Please do in this fashion for a month each meal separately. Then collect breakfast, lunch and dinner (or whatever else you may eat during the day) and self-balance for this mixture at bedtime. Then next day collect the next day's meals and self-balance before going to bed. On the third day check the first day's items and if the NST is strong you may discard it. Continue to self-balance all the items from the daily meals in this fashion for a year while you continue your regular NAET with your practitioner.

13. **Stomach acid** (Hydrochloric acid).

You may eat raw and steamed vegetables, cooked dried beans, eggs, oils, clarified butter, and milk.

14. **Base** (digestive juice from the intestinal tract contains various digestive enzymes: amylase, protease, lipase, maltase, peptidase, bromelain, cellulase, sucrase, papain, lactase, glucoamylase, and alpha galactosidase).

You may eat: sugars, starches, breads, and meats.

15. **Hormones** (estrogen, progesterone, testosterone).
You may eat vegetables, fruits, grains, chicken, and fish. Avoid red meat.
Other Hormones (histamine, endorphin, enkephalin, and acetaldehyde, growth hormone).

16. **Hypothalamus** - this part of the brain is responsible for allergic reactions in the body, especially for allergy to chemicals.

17. **Chlorox** - this is being added in various food products, herbs, spices, etc. to reduce microbial activity. This has been found one of the culprits to chemically sensitive people. Avoid everything that has chlorox or bleach in them. White flour, white fabrics (they all are bleaches), spices and herbs prepackaged by respective companies, milk, soft drinks, city water, any housecleaning products, etc.
You may eat brown rice, potato boiled with the skin (peel of the skin after boiling), cooked beef, salt, drink distilled water.

18. **Chemical mix** (chlorine, chlorox, bleach, housecleaning products, swimming pool water, detergent, fabric softener, soap,

other cleaning products, shampoos, hair products, body care products, chemicals sprays of any kind, deodorizers of any kind, lipsticks, and cosmetics you or other family members use). Avoid the contact and smell of these chemicals for 25 hours or more as tested by your NAET practitioner. In a severely sensitive person, this treatment may need to be repeated for more than a few times to achieve complete clearance. After clearing this sample test all other chemical items from your house or work that you are coming in contact with or you have contacted or used it in the past.

You may eat brown rice, potato boiled with the skin (peel of the skin after boiling), cooked beef, salt, drink distilled water.

19. Water -(drinking water, tap water, filtered water, city water, lake water, rain water, ocean water, and river water).

People can react to any water. Treat them as needed and avoid the item treated.

21. Organs (Test individual organs and if found weak treat them individually).

21. Food additives (sulfates, nitrates, BHT).

You cannot eat hot dogs or any prepackaged food. Eat anything made at home from scratch.

22. Food colors (different food colors in many sources like: ice cream, candy, cookie, gums, drinks, spices, other foods, and/or lipsticks, etc.)

You may eat foods that are freshly prepared. Avoid carrots, natural spices, beets, berries, frozen green leafy vegetables like spinach.

23. Whiten All

You may eat cooked vegetables, pasta, rice, meats, chicken, and eggs.

24. MSG (monosodium glutamate).

You may eat freshly prepared vegetables, fruits, meat, and grains without MSG.

25. Alcohol (candy, ice cream, liquid medication in alcohol, and alcohol).
You may eat vegetables, meats, fish eggs, and chicken.

26. Artificial Sweeteners (Sweet and Low, Equal, saccharine, Twin, and aspartame).

You may eat: anything without artificial sweeteners. Use freshly prepared items only.

Coffee Mix (coffee, chocolate, caffeine, tannic acid, cocoa, cocoa butter, and carob.

You may eat anything that has no coffee, caffeine, chocolate and/or carob.

Heavy metals (mercury, lead, cadmium, aluminum, arsenic, copper, gold, selenium, silver, and vanadium).

You may use only distilled water for drinking, washing and showering. You may eat only cooked rice, vegetables, fruits, meats, eggs, milk, coffee, and tea.

The items listed below are treated as needed and on a priority based protocol, which your NAET practitioner will explain to you.

Turkey (Serotonin)

You may eat any food that does not contain B1, B3, B6, tryptophane, and neurotransmitters (dopamine, epinephrine, norepinephrine, serotonin, acetylcholine).

Neurotransmitters (dopamine, epinephrine, norepinephrine, serotonin, acetylcholine).

You may eat anything other than milk products, and turkey.

Corn Mix (blue corn, yellow corn, cornstarch, corn silk, corn syrup).

You may eat only steamed vegetables, steamed rice, broccoli, baked chicken, and meats. You may drink water, tea and/or coffee without cream or sugar.

Animal Fats (body fat, butter, lard, chicken fat, beef fat, lamb fat, and fiish oil). Chemical toxins remain trapped inside the body fat cells especially in people who has allergy to fats and chemicals.

You may use anything other than the above including vegetable oils.

Vegetable Fats (corn oil, canola oil, peanut oil, linseed oil, sunflower oil, palm oil, flax seed oil, and coconut oil).

You may use steamed vegetables, steamed rice, meats, eggs, chicken, butter, and animal fats.

Vitamin F (Essential fatty acids)

You may eat anything that does not contain vegetable oils, wheat germs oils, linseed oil, sunflower oil, soybean oil, safflower oil, peanuts and peanut oil.

Spice Mix 1: (ginger, cardamom, cinnamon cloves, nutmeg, garlic, cumin, fennel, coriander, turmeric, saffron, and mint).

You may use all foods and products without these items.

Spice Mix 2 (peppers, red pepper, black pepper, green pepper, jalapeno, banana peppers, anise seed, basil, bay leaf, caraway seed, chervil, cream of tartar, dill, fenugreek, horseradish, mace, MSG, mustard, onion, oregano, paprika, poppy seed, parsley, rosemary, sage, sumac, and vinegar).

You may eat or use all foods and food products without the above listed spices.

Dried bean Mix (vegetable proteins, soybean, and lecithin).

You may eat rice, pasta, vegetables, meats, eggs, and anything other than beans and bean products.

Amino Acids-1 (essential amino acids: lysine, methionine, leucine, threonine, valine, tryptophane, isoleucine, and phenylalanine).

You may eat cooked white rice, lettuce, and boiled chicken.

Amino Acids 2 (non essential amino acids: alanine, arginine, aspartic acid, carnitine citrulline, cysteine, glutamic acid, glycine, histidine, ornithine, proline, serine, taurine, and tyrosine).

You may eat cooked white rice, boiled beef (corned beef), and iceberg lettuce.

Refined starches (corn starch, potato starch, and modified starch).

You may eat whole grains, vegetables, meats, chicken, and fish.

School work materials (crayons, coloring paper and books, inks, pencils, crayons, glue, play dough, other arts, and craft materials).
Avoid using them or contacting them. Wear a pair of gloves if you have to go near them.

Immunizations and vaccinations either you received or your parent received before you were born (DPT, POLIO, MMR, small pox, chicken pox, influenza, or hepatitis).

Any drugs given in infancy, during childhood or taken by the mother during pregnancy or taking now (antibiotics, sedatives, laxatives, or recreational drugs).

Nothing to avoid except infected persons or recently inoculated persons if there are any near you. If you treating for a drug, avoid the drug.

Fabrics (daily and sleep attire; towels, bed linens, blankets, formaldehyde, white colored clothes).

Treat each kind of fabric separately and avoid the particular cloth or kind of cloth for 25 hours.

Plastics (toys, play or work materials, utensils, toiletries, computer key boards, and/or phone).

Avoid contact with products made from plastics. Wear a pair of cotton gloves.

Perfume (room deodorizers, soaps, flowers, perfumes, or aftershave, etc.) and their smells too.
Avoid perfume and any fragrance from flowers or products containing perfume.
Check all other smells from chemicals, smoke, etc. and treat them if necessary.

Smell balancing vitamins: Molybdenum, Selenium, and Cobalt.
Nothing to avoid.

Baking powder/ Baking soda (in baked goods, toothpaste, and/ or detergents).

You may eat or use anything that does not contain baking powder or baking soda including fresh fruits, vegetables, fats, meat, and chicken.

Nothing to avoid

Nut Mix 1 (peanuts, black walnuts, or English walnuts).

You may eat any foods that do not contain the nuts listed above including their oils and butter.

Nut Mix 2: (cashew, almonds, pecan, Brazil nut, hazelnut, macadamia nut, and sunflower seeds).

You may eat any foods that do not contain the nuts listed above including their oils and butters.

Fish Mix (Cod, halibut, salmon, shark, and tuna).

You may eat any food that does not contain the fish or fish oils listed above.

Shellfish Mix (Shrimp, lobster, abalone, cray, crab, and clams).

You may eat any food that does not contain fish products.

Whey

You may eat rice, vegetables, fruits, chicken, egg, turkey, beef, pork, beans, and lamb.

Yogurt
You may eat rice, vegetables, fruits, poultry, and meat.

Gelatin
You may use anything that does not contain gelatin.

Gum Mix (Acacia, Karaya gum, Xanthine gum, black gum, sweet gum, and chewing gum).

You may eat rice, pasta, vegetables, fruits without skins, meats, eggs, and chicken, drink juice and water.

Paper Products (newspaper, newspaper ink, reading books, coloring books, books with colored illustrations, recycled paper products)

Avoid the above items.

Fluoride
You may use or eat: fruits, poultry, meat, potato, cauliflower, white rice, and yellow vegetables. You may use distilled water, drink fresh fruit juices.

Vitamin E

You may eat fresh fish, carrots, potato, poultry, and meat.

Vitamin D

You may eat fruits, vegetables, poultry, and meats.

Vitamin K

You may eat fish, rice, potato, poultry, and meat.

Night shade vegetables (bell pepper, onion, eggplant, potato, tomato (fruits, sauces, and drinks).
Avoid eating these vegetables.

Pesticides (malathion, insecticides, ant-bait, insect sprays, herbicides, termite control chemicals, regular pesticides, dioxin, fumigants, etc. and the smell from these products.)

Pesticides cause severe damages in human nervous system. Everyone involved with pesticides knows that including the scientists, researchers, manufacturers, retailers, and consumers.

Pesticides pose a real problem to chemically sensitive people causing their multiple organ system either to function inappropriately or shut down completely. This is the one of the many benefits of our scientific advantages we would like to keep because without them we would be eaten away by the pests. Chemically sensitive people must treat using NAET® all pesticides then they could prevent health hazards occurring from exposures to pesticides. This following news article was published on 08/04/06 and it clearly demonstrates the dangerous aspect of pesticides.

FRIDAY, Aug. 4 2006 (Health Day News) — Exposure to pesticides causes changes to rats' nervous systems, according to preliminary results of a project led by the Energy & Environmental Research Center (EERC) at the University of North Dakota (UND). The project seeks to identify the dangers posed by pesticides, how exposure occurs, and ways to reduce pesticide-related human health risks. In laboratory tests with rats, the researchers found that pesticide exposure caused changes in the same areas of the brain involved in multiple sclerosis, epilepsy, Parkinson's disease and Alzheimer's disease. Pesticides can also cause severe damage to the gastrointestinal system and cause neurological dysfunction, the researchers said.

Avoid meats, grasses, ant sprays, insecticides and pesticides.

Insect bites in infancy or childhood (bee stings, spider bites, or cockroach, etc.)

Treat for the individual insect and avoid it while treating.

Radiation (computer, television, microwave, X-ray, and the sun).

Avoid radiation of any kind for 25 hours following the NAET® Tx.

Inhalants

Avoid pollens, weeds, grasses, flowers, wood mix, room air, outside air, smog, and polluted air from nearby factories.

Tissues and secretions (DNA, RNA, thyroid hormone, pituitary hormone, pineal gland, hypothalamus, or brain tissue, liver, blood, and saliva).

Virus mix - Avoid people with any infections. Eat and drink freshly, well cooked foods and boiled cooled water for 24 hours following the treatment.

Bacteria mix - Avoid people with any infections. Eat and drink freshly, well cooked foods and boiled cooled water for 24 hours following the treatment.

Parasite mix - Avoid people with any infections. Eat and drink freshly, well cooked foods and boiled cooled water for 24 hours following the treatment.

Formaldhyde - Avoid things with formaldehyde.: pressed wood, dry wall, new building materials, ice cream, labels of ready made clothes, and stay awa from laboratories. Avoid touching or coming near them. Wear gloves, masks, gowns if necessary for 25 hours.

Latex products (shoe, sole of the shoe, elastic, rubber bands, and/ or rubber bathtub toys and the smells of these items).

Avoid latex products for 25 hours following the NAET® Tx.

Crude oil/Synthetic materials - Avoid them for 25 hours following the NAET® Tx.

Animal epithelial/dander - Avoid them. Avoid wool products and avoid human hair for 25 hours following the NAET® Tx. Wear gloves.

Freedom From Chemical Sensitivities

Smoking/Nicotine - avoid nicotine, tobacco and smells from the items.

Dust/Dust mites - Avoid dust for 25 hours following the NAET® Tx.

Allergies to people, animals and pets (mother, father, care takers, cats, and dogs).

Avoid the ones you were treated for 25 hours.

Emotional allergies - check all other emotional blockages and treat them with NAET® when it is needed. You may use the following list to test the emotional blockages.

Nothing to avoid for emotional treatment.

After clearing the allergy to nutrients, appropriate supplementation with vitamins, minerals, and enzymes etc., is necessary to make up the deficiency and promote healing. Please read the guidebook for information on how to take supplement correctly.

Your NAET doctor will also do a few energy boosting techniques with vitamin B complex, calcium, vitamin F, neurotransmitters, sugar, trace minerals, and magnesium.

Other chemical agents

Acetic acid

After-shave

Air freshener

Ammonia

Arsenic

Benzene

Bleach

Blood

Bottled drinking water (Check each time when you buy a new batch)

Braces & retainers

Cadmium

Carbon dioxide

Carbon monoxide

Carpet

Cat liter

Chlorine

Cigar smoke

Cleaning materials

Cleaning products

Copying ink

Correction fluids

Cosmetics you or other family members use

Detergents

Dioxin - (newspaper, paper products, bleaches, pesticides,)

EDTA)

Ethylene gas

Fabric softener

Formic acid

Fire smoke

Flea collars

Florescent light

GABA

Histamine

Household cleaning products

Ice cream

Jewelry

Jewelry cleaning solution

Lipstick

Liquid paper

Malic acid

Markers

Nickel

Nicotine

Ozone

PBDE (Polybromodiphenyl ethers

PCB (Polychlorinated biphenyls

Phenolics

Plastics-soft & hard

Polish

Polysorbate

Parasympathetic nerves

Room deodorizers

Salicylates

Shampoo

Silver

Skin creams

Smell of cigarette

Smells from chemicals

Smog

Smoking

Soap

Soda pop-cans

Serotonin

Sulfites

Swimming pool water

Sympathetic nerves

Talc

Tartaric acid

The smell of coffee brewing

The smell of popcorn

The smell of bleach or other chemicals

The smell of cigaret smoking

The smell of perfume or flowers

Tobacco

Triglycerides

Wall pictures

Water chemicals

Water pollutants

Weed-killer

Whiteout

Wood smoke

Perfume mix: all types of perfume including the smell.

Amphetamine(Speed)

Cocaine

Ecstasy

Hashish

Heroin

LSD

Magic Mushroom

Marijuana

Nicotine

Opium

PCP

Personal clothing: Pant, Shirt, Undergarments, nylons, wool, night time clothing, sanitary napkins, bed linen, bed, mattress, leather belt, leather bag, shoes, slippers, toothpaste, mouth wash.
Cosmetics, after shave, makeup, lipstick, body lotion, perfume, antiperspirant, soap, detergent and smell from these items.

Smoke: cigarette, tobacco, wood smoke, fireplace smoke, smog, sugar cane field smoke, any other kind of smoke primary or secondary in origin, smell.

Crude oil: hard plastics, soft plastics, synthetic fabrics, formaldehyde, newspaper, newspaper ink, gasoline and other products along with their smells.

TREATING BY PRIORITY

After completing the basic 15, your NAET® practitioner will evaluate your progress and if needed plan your treatment by priority to help with your immediate health problem, for example: Treating the allergen that will help with P.M.S., learning disability, dyslexia, ADHD, autism, migraine headaches, asthma, pain, etc. After the basic fifteen, the rest of the classic NAET® allergen groups can be rearranged to help with the immediate problem. This is called "treatment by priority."

All these individual treatment will work better after clearing allergies for essential nutrients— that is the NAET® Basic 15 Allergens.

Information regarding a few important acupuncture points is discussed in this chapter. They can be used to help control sensitivity reactions at any time on anyone. It is not a cure. It is going to provide temporary relief from the symptoms.

In Chapter four we learned about the twelve acupuncture meridians and their pathological symptoms when the energy circulation is blocked in those meridians (diagrams 4-1 to 4-14). In Chapter 5, using "Neuromuscular Sensitivity Testing," we learned to detect the cause of energy blockages by testing via NST for allergies. We also found that allergies may be the causative agents for energy blockages in particular meridians. We have learned to test and find the causes in general. Practice these testing techniques and make a habit of testing for everything using the self-testing procedures (if you do not have anyone else to work with you) before exposing yourself, your child or your loved one's to food, clothing, household chemicals, and environmental agents, etc., which you already know or suspect as allergens.

NAET® SELF-TESTING PROCEDURE

Hold, Sit and Test

This is the most simple allergy testing procedure (also read Chapter 3). We teach this to our patients during patient-education class. This is very simple and our young patients love it. Children are thrilled by this procedure. They test secretly for their food, cookies, drinks, clothes, etc., before the parents get to test them with NST.

Materials Needed:

1. A sample holder (thin glass jar, test tube, or a baby food jar with a lid can serve as a sample-holder).

2. Samples of the suspected allergens.

All perishable items, liquids, foods, should be placed inside the jar, then the lid should be closed tightly so that the smell will not bother the patient. If it is a piece of fabric, toy, etc., it can be held in the hand. Severe allergens like pesticides, perfume, chemicals, other toxic products should only be self-tested by adults, never by children.

Procedure:

Place a small portion of the suspected allergen in the sample holder and hold it in your palm, touching the jar with the fingertips of the same hand for 15 to 30 minutes. If you are allergic to the item in the jar, you will begin to feel uneasy when holding the allergen, giving rise to various unpleasant allergic symptoms, or exaggerating the prior allergic symptoms. The intensity of symptoms experienced is directly related to the severity of the allergy.

When one holds an allergen, one or more of the symptoms from the following list may be experienced:

Abdominal discomforts

Anger

Asthma

Backaches

Begins to get hot or cold on various parts of the body

Blurry eyes

Brain fog

Butterfly sensation in the stomach

Chest pains

Cough

Cravings

Crying spells

Deafness or ringing in the ear

Dry mouth, nose or throat

Fatigue

Flatulence

Frequency of urination

Headaches

Heaviness in the head

Heaviness in the chest

Heavy sensation in the body

Hives
Hyperactivity
Insomnia
Irregular heart beats (fast or slow)
Irritable
Itching in the nose, eyes, cheeks and ears
Knee or other joint pains
Light-headedness
Migraine headaches
Mucus in the throat
Nausea
Nervousness
Nose bleeds
Pin prick sensation
Pins and needles on the palms or soles
Poor attention span
Poor bowel control
Poor vision
Rashes
Redness on the cheeks and ears
Restlessness
Runny nose or blocked nostrils
Shortness of breath
Sinus troubles
Sneezing attacks
Sudden appearance of canker sores
Sudden eruption of acne or pimples on the face or body
Suddenly becomes silent
Suddenly becomes talkative
Unexplained pain anywhere in the body
Watering eyes
Weakness of any part of the limbs

Since the allergen is inside the sample-holder when such uncomfortable sensations are felt, the allergen can be put away immediately and the person can wash his/her hands to remove the energy of the allergen from the fingertips. This should stop the reaction immediately. In this way, you can determine allergens and the degree of allergy easily without putting yourself in danger.

SELF-BALANCING PROCEDURES

Some of the methods for self-balancing procedures are described in the following pages with appropriate diagrams for easy understanding. Please learn the procedure and practice to help you feel better.

ISOLATION TECHNIQUE

Isolating a particular blockages in a meridian can be done in many ways. One method, described here, is fairly easy to understand and with some practice this art can be mastered by anyone.

STEP 1. Balance the patient and find an indicator muscle. Refer to Chapter 5 to learn more about NST to test your allergies.
STEP 2. The patient lies down on his back with the allergen (e.g., an apple) in his resting palm. When it is needed, surrogate testing can also be used.

STEP 3. The tester touches the point in diagram 6-1 one at a time, and tests the PDM and compares the strength of the PDM in the absence and presence of the allergen. For example, touch point '1' in diagram 6-1 with the finger tips of one hand and with the other hand test the PDM, (while the patient is still holding the allergen in one hand). The muscle goes weak, indicating that the meridian or the energy pathways connected to that particular point has an energy blockage.

Point '1' (right or left) relates to the lung meridian. Obstruction in the energy flow anywhere in the lung meridian can make this point weak. Test the PDM, while touching each point in the lung meridian (for more information regarding point location in the meridians please refer to the appropriate books on acupuncture given in the bibliography). The PDM becomes the weakest when the tester touches the sites of the blocked area in the meridian. For point-meridian relationships, refer to table 6-1. Using this technique, you can trace all weak meridians and the specific weak sites in your body.

ACUTHERAPY

Acutherapy or Finger pressure therapy can be used to restore the energy flow in the blocked energy meridians temporarily.

STEP 1. The first step for finger pressure therapy is to find the organ or meridian being blocked. Find the related organ point on the table and then in the diagram 6-1.

STEP 2. When the blocked meridian is isolated, the corresponding can be point located from figure 6-1. Make the corresponding organ point as a starting point to perform the energy balancing. For example, if the energy is blocked in the liver meridian, make the liver organ point (point 5) the first point to begin the finger pressure. If the heart is blocked, use the heart point (point 2 or 3) as the first point in the sequence of energy balancing. Apply gentle but firm finger pressure with the pad of your index finger on the point. Hold 60 seconds at the first point. At the end of 60 seconds move to the next point and repeat the same. Follow the order of the sequence of points given on page 174-175.

STEP 3. Hold 60 seconds at each point and go through all 12 points and come back to the starting point. Then, hold 60 seconds at the starting point and stop the treatment. Always end at the starting point to complete the energy cycle.

Acu therapy can also help to keep your symptoms under control in these following situations:

Acute allergic reactions

Backache

Depression

Fatigue

Headache

Hyperactivity

Insomnia

Mood swings

Pain disorders

PMS (premenstrual symptoms)

Commonly seen children's disorders

It is a good idea to balance your body by applying Acu therapy or massaging the points clockwise, one minute on each points daily, twice a day. If you are very weak or sick, someone else can help to balance your points until you are strong enough to do so yourself.

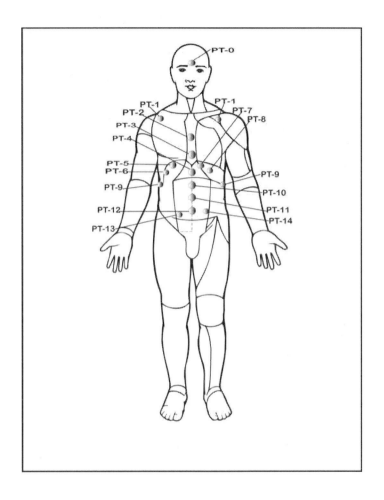

**Figure 6-1
Acutherapy Points**

POINTS TO REDUCE CHEMICAL SENSITIVITIES

You may also use general balancing points as shown in figure 6-2 to balance your body. These points in the order given in 6-2 can be massaged once or twice-a-day while you are going through NAET® treatments with a practitioner. This will help you finish the treatments easier without having to repeat multiple times for the same allergen.

You don't have to be sick to benefit from balancing the body. You can use these balancing techniques with or without NAET® treatments. Using these points you can never overbalance the body or overtreat the meridians. One can never be too healthy. If you are already healthy, you can maintain your health by doing acu therapy regularly. If you are sick, have allergies, or are unhealthy for whatever reasons, by treating these points regularly, you will feel better.

This technique can also be used in balancing the body not only in the morning or night, but any time you feel out of balance. How do you know if you are out of balance? If you are a healthy person, if your energy gets slightly out of balance you may not feel sick but may not feel quite right. You may feel tired, or sleepy in the afternoon, or not having the right motivation to do your work, etc., but you cannot find a definite reason for such "out of sorts" feeling. Some minor energy disturbance in the meridians may be the cause. If you can immediately balance the body using these points, you will clear the energy blockage and feel normal in minutes.

ACUTE CARE

If a person is having an acute health problem (e.g. shortness of breath, abdominal pain, etc.), you can use acu therapy points to help bring the problem under control. Using the same method de-

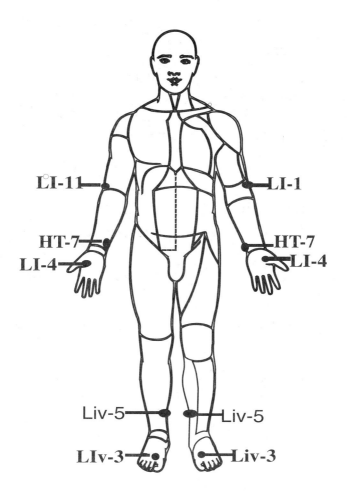

FIGURE 6-2

**POINTS TO REDUCE CHEMICAL
SENSITIVITIES**

scribed above, massage these points or emergency points often until the problem is resolved or until help arrives.

Some patients can experience physical or emotional pain or emotional release during these treatment sessions. If the patient has an emotional blockage, it needs to be isolated and treated for the best result. Some patients can get tingling pains, sharp pains, pulsation, excessive perspiration, etc. during the treatment. In such instances, please go through another cycle of treatment. Often this will correct the problem.

THE ORIENTAL MEDICINE CPR POINT

The CPR (Cardiopulmonary resuscitation) point of Oriental Medicine is the Governing Vessel-26.

Location: Below the nose, a little above the midpoint of the philtrum.

Indication: Fainting, sudden loss of consciousness, cardiac arrhythmia, heart attack, stroke, sudden loss of energy, hypoglycemia, heatstroke, sudden pain in the lower back, general lower backache, breathing problem due to allergic reactions, mental confusion, mental irritability, anger, uncontrollable rage, exercise-induced anaphylaxis, anaphylactic reactions to allergens, and sudden breathing problem due to any cause.

Procedure: Massage or stimulate the point for 30 seconds to a minute at the beginning of the problem.

• If you are treating yourself to wake up from sleeping while driving, or to recover from sudden loss of energy, etc., massage gently on this point. For example: While you are driving, if you feel sudden loss of energy or sensation of fainting, immediately massage this point. Your energy will begin to circulate faster and you will prevent a fainting episode.

• If you are reviving an unconscious victim who passed out in front of you, you may massage the point vigorously to inflict

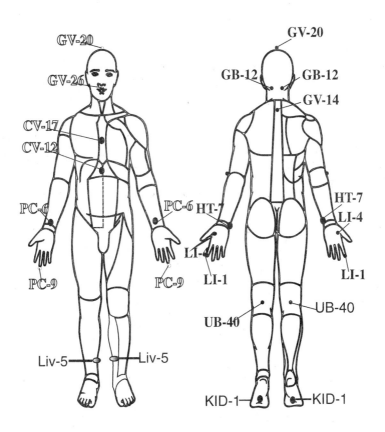

Figure 6-3

Resuscitation Points

slight pain so that the person will wake up immediately. Vigorous massage is used only to wake up the fainted person or the person who became unresponsive in front of you.

RESUSCITATION POINTS

1. Fainting: GV 26, GB 12, LI 1, PC 9
2. Nausea: CV 12, PC 6
3. Backache: GV 26, UB 40
4. Fatigue: CV 5, LI 1, CV 17
5. Fever: LI 11, LU 10, GV 16
6. Chemical sensitivity Point: LIV-5

If you see your NAET® practitioner for any acute allergic attacks (Migraine, asthma,etc.), if your practitioner is confident to treat an acute symptom, he/she may treat an allergen or a group of allergens that is suspected to be the causative agent out of the preferred order. If the practitioner is not experienced or not confident to treat an acute problem like asthma please call emergency help by calling 911 in the United States. When the acute symptom gets resolved, you can begin the NAET® treatment for the first allergen from the basic-15 list starting from the following visit. NAET® treatments can give quicker and lasting relief if done properly. If it is not done properly, you may not get the expected results.

For more information on revival techniques, refer to Chapter 3, pages 570 to 573, in "Acupuncture: A Comprehensive Text", by Shanghai College of Traditional Medicine, Eastland Press, 1981 or refer to "Living Pain Free with Acupressure" by the author. It is available at various bookstores and at our website (naet.com).

Learn these points on your body. If you have problem finding the points please ask your NAET® specialist to show them to you. Practice these techniques daily until you get perfected in doing the testing and self-balancing procedures. One or more of these emergency help points or resuscitation points can be massaged gently but firmly clockwise to help you out of most emergency situations before the emergency help arrives.

Commonly Seen emotional Blockages

Abandonment
Anger
Anxiety
Apathy
Betrayal
Bothersome
Carelessness
Concern
Confusion
Criticism
Depression
Deprivation
Despise
Disappointment
Discouragement
Disgrace
Discomfort
Disgust
Dishonor
Dislike
Distrust
Embarrassment
Envy
Failure
Faithfulness
Fear
Giving up

Grief
Guilt
Helplessness
Hopelessness
Ignore
Impatience
Insecurity
Jealousy
Loneliness
Loss
Love
Low Self Esteem
Low Self-worth
Panic
Passion
Rejection
Resentment
Sadness
Shame
Worry

7

A Collection of NAET® Cases

HOW CULLIGAN WATER FILTERING SYSTEM HELPED MY BACKACHE

I suffered from severe backaches and muscle spasms very frequently as soon as I came to Los Angeles to visit my daughter. I took analgesics, saw a chiropractor, an acupuncturist and had massages done on my back. I got some relief but the pain and muscle spasm continued to bother me. After three months staying in LA, I returned to my home in India. When I left here my back pain and muscle spasms reduced in a few hours and got complete relief in 24 hours before I reached my home. In 1984, I visited my daughter again. A day at her place my backache and back muscle spasm returned. I was dreading to come to LA because of my three-months long backache during my previous visit. By this time my daughter had made connection to illnesses with allergies. After testing me through NAET® she said I was allergic to the tap water. She treated me for the tap water and like a magic my muscle spasm and pain went away in a few minutes. I was very happy with this new treatment. My pain was gone for two days. On the third day after taking a shower I was in severe pain again. She found me reacting to water again. This time she treated me for chlorine, tap water and both combined. I got relief after treatment. But in another four days my pain and spasm returned. This pattern continued. Every three or four days my backache would return as soon as I use the water whether for washing or showering. It would be relieved after each NAET®. My daughter was puzzled too. She said that according to her theory usually after clearing the allergy to an item that item should not bother that person for rest of his/her life. It was not happening in my case on this tap water issue.

Finally she went to the water department and met with their supervisor to discuss this unique problem. There she learned that certain water chemicals are added to the city water every week depending on the need to neutralize or destroy the pollutants and contaminants they detect in the water. Water arrives in Los Angeles in an open channel from far away distance (Colorado). During its course through the open trench many contaminants like waste products, pesticides, molds, fungus, bacteria, parasites, various solvents, chemicals, soap and detergents, etc. will be mixed up in the water either fallen from the environment or thrown in by the people who live in the neighborhood. In Los Angeles, the water is collected in four different tanks to supply to different cities. Water in each tank is inspected on a regular schedule (usually once a week) for its quality and powerful chemicals like chlorine, chloramine, sodium hydroxide, ferric chloride, etc. added to the tank to destroy and neutralize the contaminants before the water department releases the water to each city then to each consumer. Each water tank is treated differently with different chemicals each time when they examine. Upon using this chemically treated water, sensitive people can have varied reactions like muscle spasms, eczema, dizziness, gastrointestinal disorders, hair loss, insomnia, etc. I suffered from all these problems but very mildly except for the backache.

Water department is aware of this problem of chemical sensitivity of certain people. If they did not treat the water and destroy the pollutants people could die from bacteria and other sources in the water. To reduce the chemical sensitivities, they do one more thing. Each city will get water supply from different tanks at several times of the month hoping to rotate the chemicals in the water supply in order to reduce the consumer's sensitivity reactions.

This explained why my NAET® treatment for the water was not holding and why I was getting my backache and other water-related health problems every three or four days. Probably those were the days they were adding new chemicals or changed the strength of the chemicals or water was supplied from different tank with different chemicals. NAET® treatments can help remove the allergy to the treated item only. When new chemicals are added or the strength of the chemicals altered, my body was seeing that batch of water as a new allergen.

My daughter started looking into installing a water filter to block out all unwanted chemicals coming into the house. After trying various filters she found Culligan water filtering system. Ever since we installed that system I have not suffered from back spasms or backache during the last thirteen years.

Sara Ambakad
La Mirada, CA

MULTIPLE CHEMICAL SENSITIVITIES

A 27 year old female presented with severe symptoms of Multiple Chemical Sensitivities causing symptoms of dizziness, brain fog, disorientation, muscle spasms, overall weakness, eyes swelling shut, throat closing up, and blackouts. She often fainted when exposed to chemical smells and was in danger of concussion from hitting her head during these sudden episodes of loss of consciousness. Smells that triggered this did not even have to be especially noxious. She had fainted at the local health food store simply from turning down the aisle where supplements and shampoos were stored. She had been experiencing these symptoms for approximately one year. She stated that: "Since the onset of MCS I have become more and more sensitized to an increasing number of chemicals. I have become virtually house-bound and have great difficulty leaving without an exacerbation of symptoms." She was unable to pursue her profession because of it. This patient treated all the basics and many other food allergies. In addition, she treated parasites, chemicals, viruses, pesticides, hormones, perfumes, mercury, plastics, formaldehyde, mold, leaf mold, and the smell of mold. She had to treat for many smells: perfumes, air freshener, bleach, fabric softener, ammonia, household cleaning products. She also treated propane, car exhaust, carpets, paint, and gasoline. We also worked on body parts: lung, adrenals, liver, gall bladder, bile, and muscles. Sometimes she didn't pass her treatments on the first try but would usually pass the next time. This patient made considerable progress. Her fainting stopped and she was able to go out in the world again. She was able to take several long trips on airplanes. At the point she moved out of state, she was much stronger and able to function much more normally again. I know she could not have made these improvements without NAET®.

NAET Sp: Sue Anderson, D.C.
Ann Arbor, MI.

M.C.S - CASE STUDY

First of all let me say thank-you, Dr. Nambudripad for giving me back my life! I have been totally disabled by Multiple Chemical Sensitivities (M.C.S.) for over a year and up until quite recently, I could not go out in public without a protective mask on. I have only had 23 treatments so far but my results have been miraculous. Perfume seemed to have been my worst problem because after that treatment I was able to take off my mask and go back out in public. I have been visiting in the homes of friends and family that I had not been able to for years. I even accompanied my husband to the mall to go for grocery shopping last weekend without any ill effects!

I felt like a child exploring all my new found freedom!

Thank-you.
Bonita Poulin
Ottawa, Canada

MIRACLE IN THE MOUNTAINS

For the past 16 years I have suffered with multiple chemical sensitivities and food allergies that have progressively gotten worse.

It has been extremely challenging for my husband Roc (who has been a great support during difficult times) and I.

Before my illness exercise was a huge part of my life. I was the picture of health as a fitness instructor, marathon runner, cross-country bicyclist, and competitive golfer. Then in 1988 after attending my husband's company picnic I became very ill and was taken to the emergency room with extreme gastrointestinal problems. After several hours I was diagnosed with a bacterial infection and sent home with antibiotics. Since that night my life has never been the same.

After seeing numerous medical doctors and specialists plus many rounds of antibiotics, I turned to holistic and alternative practitioner's who at least listened and had a more caring attitude. I've had all the mercury removed from my mouth along with detoxification programs, cleanses, diets, supplements and herbs. I eat organic and read everything I can relating to my health issues. You name it, and I've probably tried it. During some of these programs my health would improve for a while, but it would never last. I have been searching and hoping for years to find the answer to this debilitating situation.

I started NAET® treatments about 5 months ago after a friend recommended Dr. Chernoff. My health began to improve. Two months after my first treatment, my husband accepted a position in Angel Fire, New Mexico (a mountain community) that is 2 1/2 hours from our home in Santa Fe. The position came with our use of an 18-month-old furnished log home sitting at 10,000 ft. in elevation. We would be living in the house during the week then home to Santa Fe on the weekends. Although I was excited about the opportunity for Roc in this position, I was concerned about residing in this house because of my long-standing chemical sensitivities especially to new homes. Years ago I had to leave my real estate business because of my severe symptoms to building materials, etc.

Dr. Chernoff could detect and clear me on whatever she found I was allergic to in the house, and after treatments I knew that I would be able to stay there symptom free. Prior to staying a night in the house, Dr. Chernoff treated me for pesticides, teflon, and formic acid. She also needed a sample of the air in the house. Before I could get the air sample, I decided (because I was missing my husband), I would try staying in the house. I lasted 12 hours with Roc driving me home in the middle of the night. He said it was either the emergency room or home. I was in extremely bad shape. A few of my symptoms were heart palpitations, difficulty breathing, severe sinus congestion with migraine type headache, my throat was swollen and felt like it was closing, my body was swollen, red and ached. I was very confused plus I couldn't stop crying.

The next morning in Santa Fe, I was still not in great shape, but at least the crying had stopped. I called Nancy at Dr. Chernoff's office and the next few weeks I was cleared on soybeans, potato, wood mix, linseed oil, zinc, wood smoke, leather, and of course the air sample from the house. After all these treatments Dr. Chernoff said, "Now go stay in the house, and you will be fine."

It was truly astonishing the next week, but I had no symptoms coupled with the fact that I didn't smell the strong odor of linseed oil, leather, wood, eucalyptus or carpet, all of which were so intrusive just two weeks before.

There is no possible way I could have ever stayed in that house without Dr. Chernoff and the NAET treatments. Because of Dr. Chernoff's dedication, ability, knowledge of NAET plus her own personal gift as a medical intuitive, I am able to share this beautiful place in the mountains with my husband. She has a tremendous joy seeing her patients improve and return to full lives. Everyday I am improving. I have energy and am hiking 4 miles in the mountains several times a week. My mind is getting clearer and clearer plus I wake up in the morning feeling great, not tired and toxic.

Dr. Chernoff also eliminated a pain I had in my right side for 15 years. The pain is gone.

Roc and I can now travel and not worry about my sensitivity to chemicals in hotel rooms. I can shop in the mall without being sick for days or enjoy a dinner out without reacting to pesticides, perfumes etc. in restaurants.

Roc and I thank you Dr. Chernoff and NAET.

Kathryn Disario

Santa Fe, NM

THE ULTIMATE TECHNIQUE

I have been especially impressed with the use of NAET in eliminating food allergies. We have seen people who had to avoid certain foods for years such as chocolates, nuts, tomatoes, etc. who can eat these items comfortably after being cleared on them with NAET®. This is especially remarkable when we consider that conventional allergists recommend that persons with food allergies should avoid the allergic substances for the remainder of their lives. One young man had been afflicted with severe reactions to crab meat for years, and would have to eat non-seafood items when his family went to a traditional all-you-can-eat crab broil around Thanksgiving each year. After he received NAET® clearing for seafood, I saw him at a family gathering about a month later and asked how his NAET treatment was holding up. He said, "I've been making up for ten years of lost time." I like to think of NAET® as the ultimate technique for dealing with food allergies.

NAET Sp: Robert Prince, M.D.
Charlotte, North Carolina

KITTENS - CASE STUDY

Dear Dr. Devi,

My mom brought home some new kittens. Not long after I got them my legs started to get weak. After a couple weeks I could not stand up. I had to go crawling to my mom's room on my hands and knees. It was very scary. I was so scared, I thought I wasn't going to be able to walk again. My mom said maybe it is an allergy to something and called you. You said that it was my allergy to cats doing it. According to your advice, my mom got some of the cat's hair, the cat's spit, and treated me with them and in about two days, I could walk again.

Thank you so much; if it weren't for you I probably would not be walking right now. Thank you SO SO SO SO MUCH!!

Love,
Devon (9 years old)
California

CARBON MONOXIDE POISONING

I witnessed a miracle in my office today. A 74 year old lady came in for her first visit complaining of "severe acute osteoarthritis". She was having severe joint pain in her shoulders, arms, hands, and neck of 6 weeks duration. She was unable to move her arms at all without great pain and difficulty. She could not even reach out to shake my hand when I met her. She has been unable to dress herself or comb her hair recently so her children have been assisting her. If she tried to gesture while speaking or move her arms in any way she would grimace and sometimes even cry out in pain.

This all started 6 weeks ago about the same time it was discovered that she had a leaky furnace at home and had been the victim of carbon monoxide poisoning. The furnace was fixed so there has been no more exposure to carbon monoxide but this severe pain and inability to move had been with her continuously since that time.

Last week she was supposed to come in to see me for her initial visit but her pain was so severe that her son cancelled the appointment and made her go to the emergency room (against her wishes). Emergency room doctors diagnosed her with a severe acute episode of osteoarthritis and told her to take pain medication. She tried to tell them that she had never had arthritis before and that she felt there was a connection to the CO poisoning but they dismissed this and told her it was unrelated. This made her furious because she did not have any sign of arthritis until this incident and doctors refused to believe her. They tried to convince her that she must be diabetic. She's not. They also couldn't believe that when asked to list what medications she's on she said, "None." Someone her age on NO medication? They couldn't believe her! But she's a very healthy lady and has always taken care of herself and never gone to doctors. She has never had joint pain or arthritis in her life — until this incident. So she left there disgusted.

Her daughter, who is our patient, brought her in today. I told her I believed that the CO poisoning probably was related to her pain but we would have to test to find out for sure. There was no way this woman could muscle test in the shape she was in. I used her daughter as a surrogate. The patient could barely reach out to touch her daughter's hand she was in so much pain. Testing revealed that she wasn't really a very allergic person. She was OK on the first few basics. This verified what she had told me about always being healthy up until this incident.

She was very weak with the CO capsule, and NST focused this allergy was the source of her pain. The NST also focused that I could treat her for CO today as an acute condition. I treated her through her daughter. Every meridian was blocked in the presence of CO. I balanced each one of them individually with CO.

When she stood up immediately after the treatment she said she felt very different. As she walked to the next room she remarked that her arms were feeling better and she could take a deep breath for the first time in a long time. After gate points and resting, she stated that her arms had loosened up and she could move them again without pain. She started showing me that she could indeed move her arms and hands. She was astonished. By the time she walked out to the reception area she was waving her arms around and gesturing wildly, laughing, smiling, and without pain. I have seen a lot of great results with NAET® treatments before, but even I was shocked at the difference. Needless to say, she and her daughter left my office very happy. Dr. Devi, thank you for giving me the tools to help this woman today. NAET® is truly amazing.

NAET Sp:. Dr. Sue Anderson
Ann Arbor, Michigan

ENVIRONMENTALLY ILL

Thank you for giving me my life back. It's been twelve years since we had an exterminator spray our home with toxic pesticides. My body began reacting to all chemicals - I was "environmentally ill." After moving from Chicago to Taos, New Mexico seven years ago, my health improved 60%. 1 avoided all man-made chemicals, ate only organic foods and lived a very careful life-style. We recently moved to Albuquerque and I had a difficult time adjusting to our twelve year-old home - it wasn't my "adobe safe house." After treating me for the air inside and outside my house with NAET®, my whole body relaxed and I was myself again. I can sleep in a carpeted bedroom again! In fact, I was better than I had been in twelve years! I felt lighter, calmer and more focused. Amazing!

With each successive NAET® treatment, I keep getting better. I am excited about the future and the opportunity to really live life again.

Thank you, with love,
Louise Swartwalter, NM

Allergic to Cotton
"I was allergic to cotton, the kind that is in men's socks. No wonder my feet and legs ached all the time."

-Chris Kudallur
Buena Park, CA

THE END OF MY SENSITIVITIES

Dear Dr. Prince

I wanted to take a moment to thank you, your staff and NAET® for helping to restore my life to a state of excellent health.

For the past decade, I've had growing problems with food and environmental allergies. Several times a week, I would suffer from severe overall muscle pain and debilitating headaches. These episodes would last for hours and sometimes days.

After clearing the basic ten and a few other allergens with NAET®, these episodes drastically diminished in intensity and frequency. After a few more treatments, they disappeared completely. I haven't had muscle pain or headaches now for over three months. In addition, NAET® has had a positive impact on my energy level. My sinus problems, skin irritation and brain fog have also nearly disappeared.

NAET® is a wonderful discovery and you and your staff have expertly applied its techniques. I'm certain the helpful, friendly and positive manner of everyone in your office has also had a healing effect.

Thank you again for your dedication and for your marvelous work helping those of us with allergies.

Gratefully,

John Brock

NAET® SP: Dr. R. M. Prince
NAET® of Carolina

ALLERGY TO PERFUME

Wendy W., a 44 year old assistant superintendent of education and doctoral student, could not tolerate the scent of perfume, cologne or even certain flowers without getting migraine headaches. As this was a common exposure at work related meetings and classes, she was often forced to leave work or class due to the severity of her pain. After two treatments for perfume mix, Wendy states that while she still "feels" the perfume, she has had no migraines, and has not missed work or class since, due to migraine.

An interesting side note to Wendy's story involves an earlier treatment we did for chocolate. Neither she nor I thought anything about the results of that treatment until one of her co-workers complained that Wendy never had any chocolate in her desk any more. It seemed that this person could at any time find a large supply of chocolate in Wendy's drawer, and help herself. After her treatment, Wendy's craving for chocolate gradually subsided, her stash dwindled and eventually ran out without her taking notice. Sometimes an allergy can cause a craving. This type of craving reduction is not uncommon after eliminating the allergy.

Wendy's friend Debbie, also a school superintendent and attorney had been my patient for the last few moths. She began to complain of numbness in the index finger and thumb of her right hand. Myofascial release and other treatments wasn't helping. About that time I learned NAET®. I tested using my new learned skill NAET®-NST. This new test revealed that Debbie's numbness was NOT a physical problem (such as carpal tunnel syndrome), but rather a chemical/nutritional allergy.

Further NST testing showed that the allergy was to lemon Ricola cough drops she had taken 6 weeks prior. Treating twice for the cough drops (15 minutes apart) ended the numbness.

NAET® is awesome! Thank you for sharing it with us! We have a 100% NAET® practice now.

NAET® Sp: J.and M. Chianese

CHEMICALS FROM PRINTING SHOP

A 43-year-old female: Beginning about 10 years ago, she worked approximately 2 years in a print and copy shop, handling hazardous chemicals, without being provided warning or appropriate handling instructions. Her health declined during her employment there, to the point she was barely able to function. Then she accidentally found one of the warning papers, shipped with the chemicals she was using. Recognizing this was causing her health problems, she quit the job. However, her health continued to decline to the point she was house bound, and required assistance anytime she left her bed.

Seeking medical help brought the denial of her illness, or chemical toxicity, and she was told her troubles were psychosomatic or of psychogenic origin.

She turned to alternative helps, and found a naturopath and some chiropractors, who were knowledgeable and over a period of about 8 years made enough recovery to be able to move around (by using a lot of determination and rather severe self discipline). She began NAET® on October 22nd, 1999. Because of her condition, she couldn't tolerate or afford frequent treatments, but has received about 6 NAET® treatments per month for 8 months. Her recovery has not been swift, smooth or steady. Priority has been dictated repeatedly by required emergency care. Notable, was the time in March of 2000, when a radiator hose broke on her car, exposing her to ethylene glycol (anti-freeze) vapor. This made her sick and in pain for several days, and was severe enough she had to be treated through a surrogate the first two times. Definite recovery intervals were noted after the basic 10, parasites, perfume, and certain combinations from her environment.

Now, definable improvement is certain in her case. Her improvement has enabled her to secure a job, and she displays better energy, a better smile and greater hope. She appreciates us and the improvements won through NAET®.

NAET® Sp: Frank Smith, D.C..
KS

ALLERGY TO SLIM FAST

C.D., a 42 year old female, employed as a homemaker, complained of back pain getting more severe as time went on for the past few months. MRT showed an allergy to Slim Fast, which she had started taking a few months prior. She had already been treated for the basics up to Sugar Mix, so I treated her for Slim Fast and by that evening her back pain had disappeared.

NAET® SP: Cheryl Cameron,
New Brunswick, CANADA

ANT SPRAY ON THE NEWSPAPER?

On my drive back from Denver, my husband and I decided to swap driving. As we took off from the rest stop, my husband decided to read USA Today. Upon his opening the first section, I smelled a familiar odor. It wasn't the normal ink smell, but one common to the spray, RAID for ants. Immediately I asked him to put the paper away, he carefully put it behind his seat.

Since I was the designated driver, I started to get very tired behind the wheel. It must have started within 15 minutes, and I began yawning over and over, and it was very difficult to keep my eyes open. Within about forty minutes I asked him to take over. Shortly after, I fell into a deep sleep and started to feel this pain in my forehead, which became stronger and stronger. I commented that my head hurt. I started with some chest pain over my heart and the feeling of being nauseated. I definitely knew something was wrong.

We arrived back in Albuquerque and found the closest store to dispose of this paper, and to remove a small corner of the front section to get myself treated later. In checking I realized that these papers were delivered to the hotel where we were staying. At some time in transit, the vehicle or the newspaper building had to have been sprayed for ants. The paper must have been put directly on the substance and absorbed the toxins.

All I can say, a reaction can happen to anyone! And to think, that a life saving technique, NAET, can change the blocked energy field so the reaction is over and life can become normal again.

NAET Sp: Dr. Marilyn Chernoff
Albuquerque, NM

ALLERGY RELIEF, FINALLY!

I am a super fair-skinned, green-eyed, redhead who has had environmental allergies all my life. I had gone through all the "usual" allopathic tests and treatments over the years to no avail. While I was allergic to such things as tree bark, etc., no food allergies had ever been identified. I clearly remember, years ago, when I had to go off my medication for three days, "to be able to get good readings for more scratch tests"—I went into anaphylactic reactions and had to be rushed to the Emergency Room—before the three days were even up. At that point the allergist told me NEVER to go off the meds to get more tests! Guess I scared him as badly as I did myself. So, despite aggravating my asthma, I have had to live on three or more 50 milligrams doses of Benadryl for years. Talk about "dragging" myself through life. In the past two years I really got very toxic and was having severe allergic reactions to all kinds of new things that I could not identify/avoid—despite taking the Benadryl, etc. The past 8 months it got so bad that weekly I was having episodes of my eyes being so swollen that I could not see to drive. Sometimes it was one eye, sometimes the other eye, and sometimes both eyes. Then on other occasions, my lips and mouth would swell so badly, I looked like I had been beaten up—after having nothing more than water to eat/drink. Finally it got so bad that, in addition to the sporadic swelling in my eyes and face, almost every day I developed hives, bigger than the palms of my hand, ALL over my body. From scalp to arms, legs, torso and soles of my feet. I was miserable with unbearable itching and felt and looked like a monster. I also had black and blue marks everywhere from unintentional scratching during my restless, semi-sleeping nights. During both May and July I ended up being rushed in for emergency treatments for anaphylactic reactions, because my throat suddenly swelled so badly that I could not breath. Since I regularly travel on international business, I was terrified of being on a long flight when something like this might occur with no warning. When I went to work in Italy for the month of June, I carried TWO Epi-Pens, "just in case" I needed to do a self-injection of epinephrine. To confuse matters even more, I continued to get all of these allergic reactions, no matter where I traveled in the country or world. I also do medical-technical writing for inclusion in Peer Review Journals, the National Library of Medicine and Unified Medical Language System, etc. My good friend Dr. Gary Erkfritz, of Thousand Oaks, CA brought Dr. Devi's work and NAET® to my attention. I read her research results with much interest. She and I were able to work together to develop NAET®-specific insurance billing codes and get them included into a new system that is currently before the Federal Government. In July, after presenting at the NAET® Symposium, I stayed on in California and was diagnosed with about 37 severe food allergies. I went through the "basic ten" with Mala. I had some "reactions" that Mala addressed immediately, but nothing so severe as the previous breathing difficulties and swelling of my face. After completing 10 treatments, I still got hives on several occasions during the first two weeks. But, I was thrilled, that they were then only dime-sized, and not nearly so many. During the following weeks, even those episodes spaced out significantly. Now it has been over three weeks since I have had any allergy symptoms at all! And it is also over three weeks since I have had to take any Benadryl OR use my asthma inhaler. It feels so good to not be all drugged out on antihistamines, for the first time in at least 25 years. Another "side-effect" is that the swelling in my joints is now so minimal, all my rings are too big. Also, due to severe arthritis in my hips, for the last 10 years I would have to change sleeping positions at least every 30 minutes, because I would ache so badly. Now, I am only being awakened every 2-3 HOURS! Finally, some restful sleep!

A funny story. I have never been diagnosed as being allergic to dogs, (cat dander, YES!) and have had them as pets for years. I never even broke out when one licked me, etc. either. That was until I got my wonderful golden lab, Beau about 5 years ago! Whenever he would touch my skin with his nose, or heaven forbid, actually lick me, I would break out in a giant hive wherever he touched. None of my former canine friends nor my other dog, Siagi, provoked this reaction. Yet with Beau, I got gigantic hives, every single time, despite immediately washing with soap and water. So, while I was not even treated for his saliva, another very pleasant "side-effect" to the basic ten treatments is I am no longer allergic to whatever was in his spit. I leave at the end of this week to work in Poland and the UK for a month. It is the first time in years that I am not very nervous about the trip and being out of the country for an extended period of time. While I WILL carry my inhaler and Epi-pen with me, I feel certain I will not have to use either. Many, many, many thanks to Drs. Devi and Mala, Mohan and Janna!

Judy Lee, CPM, RM
New Mexico

VITAMIN C INDUCED BODY ACHE!

Tina, a thirty-year-old, complained of generalized body ache since four years. She was being treated for fibromyalgia syndrome. She stated that she ached all over her body all the time. She had no relief in spite of taking all the pain medications and numerous supplements. She also suffered from severe insomnia due to her nagging body ache. After receiving a treatment for BBF, she said she had 50% relief of her pain. After she was treated for vitamin C, her fibromyalgia disappeared. On her next visit, she brought a bottle of special brand of vitamin C from home and said that she began taking this special vitamin C exactly four years ago.

NAET® SP: Gina D' Carlo, D.C.
San Clemente, CA

NAET® MADE LIVES WORTH LIVING

I have been using NAET ®in my practice for the past 5-6 years. At first, I was somewhat skeptical: after all, how could such a simple treatment have such dramatic results when other, more traditional and accepted treatments have been unsuccessful. However, it is impossible to deny the efficacy of something that has allowed a 34 year old, severely asthmatic man to play with cats for the first time in his life without a trace of previous problem. Or allow a 5-year-old boy who was allergic to everything before allow to eat like a normal child now rather than to break out in hives when most foods touched his lips. Even more dramatically, NAET® helped a 6-year-old 'autistic' girl who was unable to speak, play or join others - her own age, in normal children's activities. I am convinced and so are my patients. Over 80% of my practice is NAET® now.

I have known Dr. Devi for twenty-five years, since our mutual days in chiropractic and acupuncture schools. She has made a lasting impression on the lives of thousands of people, and I am proud to be associated with her. I enjoy doing NAET® and solving many puzzles of my difficult patients with their so called incurable health problems. I will continue to help as many people as I can with this simple, direct and effective system that she developed. Dr. Devi is changing lives and making some lives worth living; what can be more rewarding and worthwhile than that?

Susan Meisinger D.C., L.Ac.
Woodland Hills, CA

I HANDLED MY WEIGHT PROBLEM
THROUGH NAET®

I began gaining weight in my late teens. I continued to gain about 10 pounds every year ever since. I tried everything I could think of to get my weight down, including 10 different diet plans through the years. I barely ate to live, yet my pounds didn't go down. The more careful I got the more I just continued to pack pounds. It was awful. It was disgusting, depressing, I even tried yeast-free diets, thyroid, antidepressants and laxatives.... No one had any answer to my obesity.

Then I developed a severe nasal allergy. Burning and itching inside and outside my nostrils. I also developed vaginal candidiasis. Again none of the treatments I tried was working on me. It seemed that I was resistant to all types of treatments. I met a lady in a health food store. She suggested NAET®. I had no hope with

NAET® either. As a last resort, I decided to start NAET® treatments. What is there to lose?

To my surprise my practitioner found the cause of my problem on the very first visit. I was allergic to everything I ate. By the time I finished the basic NAET® treatments, I was seeing results. My nasal allergy stopped and my weight began dropping, slowly but surely. I was happy because finally something was working on me. I continued NAET® regularly, three times a week for the last three years. After about 150 NAET® treatments in my practitioner's office and many self-treatments at home, I can say that I am fairly healthy now and weigh 50 pounds less than three years ago.

Every morning I weigh myself and if I see a weight gain even if it is one pound, I muscle test (O-ring test) myself and find the food or drink I ate previous day that caused a weight gain and I self-treat every 15 minutes for 6 times before I eat anything. Thank God this is working well and keeping my weight normal and yeast infection problem completely under control for the first time in years.

Thanks again to NAET®.
Jane Jones, LA, CA

I AM ENJOYING MY LIFE AGAIN!

Dear Doctor,

I want to thank you for introducing me to NAET®. It has changed my life in so many ways. As you know, I have suffered from allergies/hay-fever since youth. I have been treated on and off for years. The most significant were shots in the late 70's to mid 80's at which time I was declared, "cured". I still had problems in the spring and fall, however. In the 90's I turned to over the counter medicines at times double and triple dosages to survive. On March 15, 1994 I started homeopathic cure process which was effective. I have not had medication since. However, I have suffered while mowing grass (headaches and wheezing) and in the spring and fall with flowering trees and falling leaves. This is all history now. I had a lot more problems that were masked by a constant congestion and ill feeling that I just got used to. Another Problem I had was my body getting used to any new environment when I traveled. Even with the homeopathic "cure" I would feel like I had a flu for a day when I would go from Boston to Minnesota (my home state) then again for a day going to visit relatives in South Dakota from there. The reverse was also true returning back. So in a one-week vacation I probably felt myself and enjoyed myself for 3-4 days, that is if there was no fresh cut grass. Well, now the rest of the story:

You introduced me to NAET®. My initial complaints were problems breathing while cutting grass and arthritis. Your first treatment was for chicken and feathers. Two days I mowed grass and for the first time without a breathing problem and residual headache. What can I say!!! Marvelous!

Let's go on: After clearing for Calcium my diagnosed (through CT scan) osteoarthritis pain in my clavicle joint started to subside to the point it is essentially gone now. As you know I could hardly get a shirt on because of the restriction and pain. After clearing the sulfur my arthritis is almost gone. After mold treatment, I was more clearheaded and freer of breathing problems.

The oak treatment again enhanced clear headedness, more focus and calmer demeanor. The most recent treatment that made the most miraculous change, namely for flowers and perfume two weeks before my mother passed away. When the flowers arrived at the funeral home I thought I would be in serious trouble. To my surprise hardly an effect... no headache or congestion, etc. Later the flowers were brought to the home, which again my body was able to adapt and have no problems or side effects. Now that we have the beautiful flowering trees which in the past ruined my spring. This is the first spring that I have enjoyed walking and enjoying the trees and beauty... no headaches, congestion, etc. I am overjoyed. I just returned from a trip to Minnesota and South Dakota. I enjoyed ever day! No getting used to the new environment each part of the trip as in the past. I love to golf in the morning, which in the spring is the worst time because of the pollen and fresh cut grass (golf courses mow the grass early in the morning). I would react to these allergens by developing neck and shoulder tightness and tension. Obviously, the worst spot on the body to ruin a golf game. That so far is no longer a problem and my golf game has improved. Finally, I had mucus build up during the night and especially bad upon getting up. That symptom is virtually gone. I can finally wear the teeth night guard that my dentist insists I wear. I could not previously wear it through the night because of my congestion which is now gone and I can now protect my teeth at night by wearing the night guard.

I have probably missed some of the other changes and look forward to Further improvements. Again thank you for your effective NAET® treatments. It has been painless and without the side effects of drugs.

Regards
Dave

NAET practitioner:
Marcia Costello, R.N., M. Ac., L.Ac.

NO MORE ANAPHYLACTIC REACTIONS

I am 44 years old and for a little over 3 years have been suffering from seafood, fish, dairy, spice, perfume, and cigarette smoke allergies.

As soon as I came in contact with one of these products, I swelled up and would have to either go to the hospital or take 3 Benadryl to prevent any more swelling. Also, whenever I ate chocolate or drank coffee, I got lumps in my left breast. I had to have a mammogram every year to make sure it was not cancerous. Ever since I had my second daughter, Céline, and got my tubes tied, I suffered from hot flashes, migraines, and my menstrual cycles was never 28 days; it was more like every 17 to 28 days. My family doctor had told me that I was going through premenopause.

After seeing the extraordinary results of Cheryl's treatments for my daughter Jessica's allergies, I made up my mind, and right after receiving the first treatment which balances your brain and your body, I never again had hot flashes, migraines, and my menstrual cycle is now every 35 days. After the 5th treatment, I could eat ice cream as well as any other dairy product. During the 9th treatment, with Cheryl present, I ate a small lobster claw with no allergic reaction and I now eat fish or seafood twice a week with no problem.

Cheryl also treated me for chocolate, coffee and caffeine and I no longer have any lumps in my breast. I can eat chocolate and drink coffee with no problems.

I recommend NAET® to all persons suffering from allergies. You will be very surprised at the very positive results you will have.

Thank you Cheryl.

Chantal Arseneau
Robertville

NAET Sp: Cheryl Cameron
North Tetagouche, NB E2A 4Y7

I WAS ANAPHYLACTIC TO SHELLFISH

I reacted severely to fish or fish products since childhood. Whenever I ate a minute portion of fish or shellfish, my throat closed up, I couldn't breathe, I would break out with huge hives all over my body and I ended up in the emergency room for hours with cortisone and other emergency drugs. On a few occasions, I had to be hospitalized for a few days. One of my friends, who was treated by Dr. Devi for his peanut allergy, suggested that I see her for my life-threatening fish allergy. I was curious about NAET. She treated me for all the basics before she treated me for fish groups.

I had a severe reaction during the first treatment for fish. As soon as she placed the clear glass vial with the energy of fish in my hand, my hand swelled up and I broke out in red hives all over my body. I got up from the treatment table to reach for my adrenaline shot which I carried all the time with me. But she stopped me. She commanded me to turn over. She looked very confident. I obeyed her and she applied firm pressure on my back, up and down along the spine for a few times. When she finished applying the acupressure along my spine, she asked me to turn on my back. She tested my arm. I was strong. She asked me how I was doing. I was breathing better than ever and my throat did not feel restricted anymore. I looked at my bare arms. Red rashes began fading away. This is magic, I thought. She was standing in front of me with that smile of confidence, waiting for my answer. "Better," I said, with a sigh of relief. I had to have three combination treatments for fish (fish group, lungs, colon, spleen and liver, fish group and base, fish group and heat, each on a separate office visit). After completion of the treatments, she told me to hold a small portion of fish in my palm and sit for 30 minutes. I felt fine. Then she asked me to eat a small portion of fish. I had my adrenaline near me when I ate a piece of fish, but nothing happened.

Ever since I was treated for fish, I eat fish at least twice a week without any problem. This is the best discovery man (woman) has ever made in medicine.

Dave Moore
Laguna Beach, California

MY CHRONIC COUGH

I suffered from severe dry cough for four years. I coughed throughout the day. It became worse at night after I would go to bed, and early in the morning when I woke up. I tried Western medicine, holistic medicine, and homeopathic remedies for four years. Nothing gave any relief. I changed my bed linen to 100% cotton, kept my home free of dust, used air and water purifiers. I tried every possible treatment known to get relief. Then I was guided to Dr. Devi by a friend. She evaluated me in her office and, on the very first visit, asked me if I was using any special mouthwash. I used this special mouthwash every night before I went to bed and every morning after I brushed my teeth. She treated me for the mouthwash. I had to avoid it for 40 hours. My cough stopped, just as if someone had turned off a switch, after the treatment for the mouthwash. Now I use it regularly without any trouble.

Marion Stills,
Costa Mesa, CA.

BRONCHIAL ASTHMA AND BODY ACHE

For approximately 15 years, I have suffered with frequent colds that turn into extended bouts with bronchial asthma and extreme weakness and fatigue. The doctors treated me with extensive doses of antibiotics, steroids, antihistamines, and cough medicine. I was usually depressed and so weak I could hardly move out of bed and had to get shots every day for weeks. Along with it, my stomach would gurgle and hurt for the duration of the medication. The doctors thought the stomach problems were due to steroids.

One night I had the flu and started wheezing, so I took some of the cough medicine I used to take. I had not had a cold since I moved out of Louisiana's humid climate, but I still had some of my old cough medicine. One hour later, I awoke, aching all over, with my stomach hurting and gurgling in that old familiar way. It brought back memories of the past when I had been so sick. I called Dr. Devi and she told me to bring the cough medicine. As soon as she treated me for it I got my strength back, was no longer depressed, and my stomach felt normal. I had continuous yeast infections for years. After being treated for toilet paper they disappeared.

When I started with Dr. Devi, I had severe body pain in my neck, head and shoulders. After being treated for the labels in my clothes (cotton and silk), the pain decreased dramatically.

Carole W.
Irvine, CA

HE WAS ANAPHYLACTIC TO PEANUTS

My eight year old son had severe peanut allergy ever since he was a baby. When he was three years old he had to be taken to the emergency room after he ate a touch of peanut butter. He would get asthma, break out in huge hives and his throat would swell if he smelled peanut oil or roasted peanuts. So we never used peanuts or peanut oil in the house. It was a nightmare for me to read all the labels before I buy food products or send him to school where children eat peanuts and candies and most of them included peanuts. Then I heard about NAET. Sam was treated by NAET for peanuts. After he was treated he accidently ate a cookie with peanut. He did not have a reaction. I am not planning to feed him peanuts for meals. But I am more at ease now knowing that he will not have a life-threatening reaction if he ate peanuts accidently somewhere. Thank you Dr. Devi, for your miraculous contribution to the world!

Sharon M.
Long Beach, CA

BELL PEPPER AND ASTHMA

I used to get asthma, indigestion and depression whenever I ate anything with bell pepper. After I was treated by Dr. Devi for the allergy to bell pepper, I was able to eat and enjoy bell peppers without getting any asthma or indigestion and depression. Since being treated for the allergy to eggs, I do not get any of the above-mentioned problems whenever I eat eggs.

Dianne M.
Los Angeles, CA

NO MORE NASAL INFECTION

Shortly after beginning a new career in interior design, I suddenly contacted a nasal infection due to allergies that, up until then, I did not realize I had. The infection worsened until I finally was operated on to keep it from spreading into the brain and to alleviate the worsening pressure, frequency and intensity of asthmatic attacks. During that seven-year period I had allergy shots, cortisone shots, antihistamines, and antibiotics prescribed by numerous medical doctors, none of which worked. The year the infection worsened before the operation, I began seeing Dr. Devi who pinpointed some major allergens. After treatment for many of them, I found I no longer reacted to those particular allergens and I started on the beginning of the healing process. However, the degree of infection up until then hampered the body's ability to respond quickly; so the operation was necessary to assist the process and halt the spreading of the infection. Almost two cups of infectious materials were removed from six packed sinus cavities.

After the operation, I had asthmatic attacks to a lesser degree, but still had not cleared the body of continuing infection, and was unable to work. When Dr. Devi began assisting in the total elimination of the infection, the accelerated healing process began. Through diligence and persistence, Dr. Devi uncovered allergens (unrecognized by conventional medicines) that I had been exposed to through my work, such as resins, and formaldehyde, which were major contributors to my illness. Of course, many foods, plants, and other chemicals contributed towards my ill health, too. But it seems that NAET actually cured the body from reacting to those particular allergens. I had the sinus surgery in 1988. I haven't had any recurrence of my sinus infections or asthmatic attacks for the past fifteen years. I did not have to give up my job as an interior decorator-designer, which I love so much. I am so fortunate to have discovered Dr. Devi and NAET.

Shirley R
Diamond Bar, CA.

I WAS ALLERGIC TO MY NASAL SPRAY

Every time I used nasal spray, my face would turn red. After NAET treatment, I could use nasal spray with no ill effects. Being asthmatic, I was taking two oral medications and using three inhalers. Since my NAET treatments from Dr. Devi for my inhalers, not only has my medication been reduced by 50%, but my oral medication has also been reduced.

Joyce Bastian
Newport Beach, CA

FEAR TRIGGERED HIS ASTHMA

Every Saturday, my seven year old son suffered from asthmatic attacks. Medication or sprays did not help him at all. I had to take him to the doctor's office or emergency room. Just by sitting in the emergency room waiting area, his asthma would go away. Saturday was his father's turn to take him for the weekend. Since he was not feeling well on Saturday night, he could not go with him. When I brought him to Dr. Devi, she found that the cause of his asthma was an emotional issue. He was afraid to go with his father because he would have to spend the night in his room with his gay roommate. So he began having asthmatic episodes, spending Saturday evening in the emergency room. Then Sunday, his father would take him out for a couple of hours. After he was treated for his allergy and fear of his father's roommate, he stopped having Saturday night asthma.

Belle Cole
Fullerton, CA

BRONCHIAL ASTHMA

A woman who suffered from bronchial asthma was cleared of her asthma when she was treated for pneumococcus, the bacterium responsible for pneumonia. Both of her parents had died of pneumonia soon after her birth.

NAET Sp: Mary Baty
Los Angeles, CA

NAET® HAS GIVEN ME MY LIFE BACK!

Dear Dr. Nambudripad,

I had severe allergies to grass, pollen, dairy, animal dander and smoke. These allergies hindered my ability to spend time out side:

Freedom From Chemical Sensitivities

Going to barbecues, going to the park with friends or even leaving my house in the spring time were terribly difficult.

Now after several NAET treatments from Dr. Lisa I have no symptoms of any asthma or allergies at all. I can play with my cat, have picnics in the park, and have back yard barbecues, and do all the things a normal teenager does without any kind of pain.

I'm so grateful to Dr. Lisa for treating me and to you for discovering this wonderful therapy.

Thank you Dr. Devi Nambudrpad
Thank you Dr. Lisa Camerino

Paul, Oregon

Glossary

Acetaldehyde: An aldehyde found in cigarette smoke, vehicle exhaust, and smog. It is a metabolic product of Candida albicans and is synthesized from alcohol in the liver.

Acetylcholine: A neurotransmitter manufactured in the brain, used for memory and control of sensory input and muscular output signals.

Acid: Any compound capable of releasing a hydrogen ion; it will have a pH of less than 7.

Acute: Extremely sharp or severe, as in pain, but can also refer to an illness or reaction that is sudden and intense.

Adaptation: Ability of an organism to integrate new elements into its environment.

Addiction: A dependent state characterized by cravings for a particular substance if that substance is withdrawn.

Additive: A substance added in small amounts to foods to alter the food in some way.

Adrenaline: Trademark for preparations of epinephrine, which is a hormone secreted by the adrenal gland. It is used sublingually and by injection to stop allergic reactions.

Aldehyde: A class of organic compounds obtained by oxidation of alcohol. Formaldehyde and acetaldehyde are members of this class of compounds.

Alkaline: Basic, or any substance that accepts a hydrogen ion; its pH will be greater than 7.

Allergenic: Causing or producing an allergic reaction.

Allergen: Any organic or inorganic substance from one's surroundings or from within the body itself that causes an allergic response in an individual is called an allergen. An allergen can cause an IgE antibody mediated or non-IgE mediated response. Some of the commonly known allergens are: pollens, molds, animal dander, food and drinks, chemicals of different kind like the ones found in food, water, inside and outside air, fabrics, cleaning agents, environmental materials, detergent, cosmetics, perfumes, etc., body secretions, bacteria, virus, synthetic materials, fumes of any sort, including pesticide fumes, fumes from cooking, etc., and smog. Emotional unpleasant thoughts like anger, frustration, etc. can also become allergens and cause allergic reactions in people.

Allergic reaction: Adverse, varied symptoms, unique to each person, resulting from the body's response to exposure to allergens.

Allergy: Attacks by the immune system on harmless or even useful things entering the body. Abnormal responses to substances that are usually well tolerated by most people.

Amino acid: An organic acid that contains an amino (ammonia-like NH3) chemical group; the building blocks that make up all proteins.

Anaphylactic shock: Also known as anaphylaxis. Usually happens suddenly when exposed to a highly allergic item. But sometimes, it can also happen as a cumulative reaction. (first two doses of penicillin may not trigger a severe reaction, but the third or fourth could produce an anaphylaxis in some people). An anaphylaxis (this life threatening allergic reaction) is characterized by: an immediate allergic reaction that can cause difficulty in breathing, light headedness, fainting, sensation of chills, internal cold, severe heart palpitation or irregular heart beats, pallor, eyes rolling, poor mental clarity, tremors, internal shaking, extreme fear, angio neurotic edema, throat swelling, drop in blood pressure, nausea, vomiting, diarrhea, swelling anywhere in the body, redness and hives, fever, delirium, unresponsiveness, or sometimes even death.

Antibody: A protein molecule produced in the body by lymphocytes in response to a perceived harmful foreign or abnormal substance as a defense mechanism to protect the body.

Antigen: Any substance recognized by the immune system that causes the body to produce antibodies; also refers to a concentrated solution of an allergen.

Antihistamine: A chemical that blocks the reaction of histamine that is released by the mast cells and basophils during an allergic reaction. Any substance that slows oxidation, prevents damage from free radicals and results in oxygen sparing.

Assimilate: To incorporate into a system of the body; to transform nutrients into living tissue.

Autoimmune: A condition resulting when the body makes antibodies against its own tissues or fluid. The immune system attacks the body it inhabits, which causes damage or alteration of cell function.

Binder: A substance added to tablets to help hold them together.

Blood brain barrier: A cellular barrier that prevents certain chemicals from passing from the blood to the brain.

Buffer: A substance that minimizes changes in pH (Acidity or alkalinity).

Candida albicans: A genus of yeast like fungi normally found in the body. It can multiply and cause infections, allergic reactions or toxicity.

Candidiasis: An overgrowth of Candida organisms, which are part of the normal flora of the mouth, skin, intestines and vagina.

Carbohydrate, complex: A large molecule consisting of simple sugars linked together, found in whole grains, vegetables, and fruits. This metabolizes more slowly into glucose than refined carbohydrate.

Carbohydrate, refined: A molecule of sugar that metabolizes quickly to glucose. Refined white sugar, white rice, white flour are some of the examples.

Catalyst: A chemical that speeds up a chemical reaction without being consumed or permanently affected in the process.

Cerebral allergy: Mental dysfunction caused by sensitivity to foods, chemicals, environmental substances, or other substances like work materials etc.

Chronic: Of long duration.

Chronic fatigue syndrome: A syndrome of multiple symptoms most commonly associated with fatigue and reduced energy or no energy.

Crohn's disease: An intestinal disorder associated with irritable bowel syndrome, inflammation of the bowels and colitis.

Cumulative reaction: A type of reaction caused by an accumulation of allergens in the body.

Cytokine Immune system's second line of defense. Examples of cytokines are interleukin 2 and gamma interferon.

Desensitization: The process of building up body tolerance to allergens by the use of extracts of the allergenic substance.

Detoxification: A variety of methods used to reduce toxic materials accumulated in body tissues.

Digestive tract: Includes the salivary glands, mouth, esophagus, stomach, small intestine, portions of the liver, pancreas, and large intestine.

Disorder: A disturbance of regular or normal functions.

Dust: Dust particles from various sources irritate sensitive individual causing different respiratory problems like asthma, bronchitis, hay-fever like symptoms, sinusitis, and cough.

Dust mites: Microscopic insects that live in dusty areas, pillows, blankets, bedding, carpets, upholstered furniture, drapes, corners of the houses where people neglect to clean regularly.

Eczema: An inflammatory process of the skin resulting from skin allergies causing dry, itchy, crusty, scaly, weepy, blisters or eruptions on the skin. skin rash frequently caused by allergy.

Edema: Excess fluid accumulation in tissue spaces. It could be localized or generalized.

Electromagnetic: Refers to emissions and interactions of both electric and magnetic components. Magnetism arising from electric charge in motion. This has a definite amount of energy.

Elimination diet: A diet in which common allergenic foods and those suspected of causing allergic symptoms have been temporarily eliminated.

Endocrine: refers to ductless glands that manufacture and secrete hormones into the blood stream or extracellular fluids.

Endocrine system: Thyroid, parathyroid, pituitary, hypothalamus, adrenal glands, pineal gland, gonads, the intestinal tract, kidneys, liver, and placenta.

Endogenous: Originating from or due to internal causes.

Environment: A total of circumstances and/or surroundings in which an organism exists. May be a combination of internal or external influences that can affect an individual.

Environmental illness: A complex set of symptoms caused by adverse reactions of the body to external and internal environments.

Enzyme: A substance, usually protein in nature and formed in living cells, which starts or stops biochemical reactions.

Eosinophil: A type of white blood cell. Eosinophil levels may be high in some cases of allergy or parasitic infestation.

Exogenous: Originating from or due to external causes.

Extract: Treatment dilution of an antigen used in immunotherapy, such as food, chemical, or pollen extract.

Fibromyalgia: An immune complex disorder causing general body aches, muscle aches, and general fatigue.

"Fight" or "flight": The activation of the sympathetic branch of the autonomic nervous system, preparing the body to meet a threat or challenge.

Food addiction: A person becomes dependent on a particular allergenic food and must keep eating it regularly in order to prevent withdrawal symptoms.

Food grouping: A grouping of foods according to their botanical or biological characteristics.

Free radical: A substance with unpaired electrode, which is attracted to cell membranes and enzymes where it binds and causes damage.

Gastrointestinal: Relating both to stomach and intestines.

Heparin: A substance released during allergic reaction. Heparin has antiinflammatory action in the body.

Histamine: A body substance released by mast cells and basophils during allergic reactions, which precipitates allergic symptoms.

Holistic: Refers to the idea that health and wellness depend on a balance between the physical (structural) aspects, physiological (chemical, nutritional, functional) aspects, emotional and spiritual aspects of a person.

Homeopathic: Refers to giving minute amounts of remedies that in massive doses would produce effects similar to the condition being treated.

Homeostasis: A state of perfect balance in the organism, also called "Yin-yang" balance. The balance of functions and chemical composition within an organism that results from the actions of regulatory systems.

Hormone: A chemical substance that is produced in the body, secreted into body fluids, and is transported to other organs, where it produces a specific effect on metabolism.

Hydrocarbon: A chemical compound that contains only hydrogen and carbon.

Hypersensitivity: An acquired reactivity to an antigen that can result in bodily damage upon subsequent exposure to that particular antigen.

Hyperthyroidism: A condition resulting from over-function of the thyroid gland.

Hypoallergenic: Refers to products formulated to contain the minimum possible allergens and some people with few allergies can tolerate them well. Severely allergic people can still react to these items.

Hypothyroidism: A condition resulting from under-function of the thyroid gland.

IgA: Immunoglobulin A, an antibody found in secretions associated with mucous membranes.

IgD: Immunoglobulin D, an antibody found on the surface of B-cells.

IgE: Immunoglobulin E, an antibody responsible for immediate hypersensitivity and skin reactions.

IgG: Immunoglobulin G, also known as gammaglobulin, the major antibody in the blood that protects against bacteria and viruses.

IgM: Immunoglobulin M, the first antibody to appear during an immune response.

Immune system: The body's defense system, composed of specialized cells, organs, and body fluids. It has the ability to locate, neutralize, metabolize and eliminate unwanted or foreign substances.

Immunocompromised: A person whose immune system has been damaged or stressed and is not functioning properly.

Immunity: Inherited, acquired, or induced state of being, able to resist a particular antigen by producing antibodies to counteract it. A unique mechanism of the organism to protect and maintain its body against adversity by its surroundings.

Inflammation: The reaction of tissues to injury from trauma, infection, or irritating substances. Affected tissue can be hot, reddened, swollen, and tender.

Inhalant: Any airborne substance small enough to be inhaled into the lungs; eg., pollen, dust, mold, animal danders, perfume, smoke, and smell from chemical compounds.

Intolerance: Inability of an organism to utilize a substance.

Intracellular: Situated within a cell or cells.

Intradermal: method of testing in which a measured amount of antigen is injected between the top layers of the skin.

Ion: An atom that has lost or gained an electron and thus carries an electric charge.

Kinesiology: Science of movement of the muscles.

Latent: Concealed or inactive.

Leukocytes: White blood cells.

Lipids: Fats and oils that are insoluble in water. Oils are liquids in room temperature and fats are solid.

Lymph: A clear, watery, alkaline body fluid found in the lymph vessels and tissue spaces. Contains mostly white blood cells.

Lymphocyte: A type of white blood cell, usually classified as T- or B-cells.

Macrophage: A white blood cell that kills and ingests microorganisms and other body cells.

Masking: Suppression of symptoms due to frequent exposure to a substance to which a person is sensitive.

Mast cells: Large cells containing histamine, found in mucous membranes and skin cells. The histamine in these cells are released during certain allergic reactions.

Mediated: Serving as the vehicle to bring about a phenomenon, eg., an IgE-mediated reaction is one in which IgE changes cause the symptoms and the reaction to proceed.

Membrane: A thin sheet or layer of pliable tissue that lines a cavity, connects two structures, selective barrier.

Metabolism: Complex chemical and electrical processes in living cells by which energy is produced and life is maintained. New material is assimilated for growth, repair, and replacement of tissues. Waste products are excreted.

Migraine: A condition marked by recurrent severe headaches often on one side of the head, often accompanied by nausea, vomiting, and light aura. These headaches are frequently attributed to food allergy.

Mineral: An inorganic substance. The major minerals in the body are calcium, phosphorus, potassium, sulfur, sodium, chloride, and magnesium.

Mucous membranes: Moist tissues forming the lining of body cavities that have an external opening, such as the respiratory, digestive, and urinary tracts.

Muscle Response Testing (MRT) or Neuromuscular testing (NST): A testing technique based on kinesiology to test allergies by comparing the strength of a muscle or a group of muscles in the presence and absence of the allergen.

NAR Foundation (NARF): A nonprofit research foundation dedicated to conduct research in allergy elimination of food, chemicals, environmental and other substances using NAET

NAET: (Nambudripad's Allergy Elimination Techniques): A technique to permanently eliminate allergies towards the treated allergens. Developed by Dr. Devi S. Nambudripad and practiced by more than 8,000 medical practitioners worldwide. This technique is natural, non-invasive, and drug-free. It has been effectively used in treating all types of allergies and problems arising from allergies. It is taught by Dr. Nambudripad in Buena Park, California. to currently licensed medical practitioners. If you are a licensed medical practitioner, interested in learning more about NAET, or NAET seminars, please visit the website: www.naet.com.

Nervous system: A network made up of nerve cells, the brain, and the spinal cord, which regulates and coordinates body activities.

NST: Neuromuscular testing (NST): A testing technique based on kinesiology to test allergies by comparing the strength of a muscle or a group of muscles in the presence and absence of the allergen.

NTT: A series of standard diagnostic tests used by NAET practitioners to detect allergies is called "Nambudripad's Testing Techniques" or NTT.

Neurotransmitter: A molecule that transmits electrical and/or chemical messages from nerve cell (neuron) to nerve cell or from nerve cell to muscle, secretory, or organ cells.

Nutrients: Vitamins, minerals, amino acids, fatty acids, and sugar (glucose), which are the raw materials needed by the body to provide energy, effect repairs, and maintain functions.

Organic foods: Foods grown in soil free of chemical fertilizers, and without pesticides, fungicides and herbicides.

Outgasing: The releasing of volatile chemicals that evaporate slowly and constantly from seemingly stable materials such as plastics, synthetic fibers, or building materials.

Overload: The overpowering of the immune system due to numerous concurrent exposures or to continuous exposure caused by many stresses, including allergens.

Parasite: An organism that depends on another organism (host) for food and shelter, contributing nothing to the survival of the host.

Pathogenic: Capable of causing disease.

Pathology: The scientific study of disease; its cause, processes, structural or functional changes, developments and consequences.

Pathway: The metabolic route used by body systems to facilitate biochemical functions.

Peakflow meter: An inexpensive, valuable tool used in measuring the speed of the air forced out of the lungs and helps to monitor breathing disorders like asthma.

Petrochemical: A chemical derived from petroleum or natural gas.

pH: A scale from 1 to 14 used to measure acidity and alkalinity of solutions. A pH of 1-6 is acidic; a pH of 7 is neutral; a pH of 8-14 is alkaline or basic.

Postnasal drip: The leakage of nasal fluids and mucus down into the back of the throat.

Precursor: Anything that precedes another thing or event, such as physiologically inactive substance that is converted into an active substance that is converted into an active enzyme, vitamin, or hormone.

Prostaglandin: A group of unsaturated, modified fatty acids with regulatory functions.

Radiation: The process of emission, transmission, and absorption of any type of waves or particles of energy, such as light, radio, ultraviolet or X-rays.

Receptor: Special protein structures on cells where hormones, neurotransmitters, and enzymes attach to the cell surface.

Respiratory system: The system that begins with the nostrils and extends through the nose to the back of the throat and into the larynx and lungs.

Rotation diet: A diet in which a particular food and other foods in the same "family" are eaten only once every four to seven days.

Sensitivity: An adaptive state in which a person develops a group of adverse symptoms to the environment, either internal or external. Generally refers to non-IgE reactions.

Serotonin: A constituent of blood platelets and other organs that is released during allergic reactions. It also functions as a neurotransmitter in the body.

Sublingual: Under the tongue–method of testing or treatment in which a measured amount of an antigen or extract is administered under the tongue, behind the teeth. Absorption of the substance is rapid in this way.

Supplement: Nutrient material taken in addition to food in order to satisfy extra demands, effect repair, and prevent degeneration of body systems.

Susceptibility: An alternative term used to describe sensitivity.

Symptoms: A recognizable change in a person's physical or mental state, that is different from normal function, sensation, or appearance and may indicate a disorder or disease.

Syndrome: A group of symptoms or signs that, occurring together, produce a pattern typical of a particular disorder.

Synthetic: Made in a laboratory; not normally produced in nature, or may be a copy of a substance made in nature.

Systemic: Affecting the entire body.

Target organ: The particular organ or system in an individual that will be affected most often by allergic reactions to varying substances.

Toxicity: A poisonous, irritating, or injurious effect resulting when a person ingests or produces a substance in excess of his or her tolerance threshold.

One of my patients sent the following and wanted to know if I thought these symptoms had anything to do with allergies since I have told often that there is an allergy as an underlying factor in most human illnesses. Yes, of course, I think the people suffering from these symptoms may qualify to call themselves as chemically sensitive or say suffering from multiple chemical sensitivities. I have treated a few of such problems in the past successfully. So I decided to look at these problems through the eyes of NAET and came up possible allergies to most of these problems. If anyone is suffering from these disorders try to test these suggested items and see if you find any abnormal sensitivities to them. If you detect your allergies then you have a way to eliminate them now through NAET.

LITTLE KNOWN SYNDROMES THAT ARE REAL

AIR CONTROLLERS SYNDROME:
Peptic ulcers occurring among air traffic controllers, as a result of job stress. {Illinois Medical Journal, 1972}

(Allergy to calcium, B vitamins. Treat with NAET and take supplements for a while)

ALOPECIA WALKMANIA:
Loss of hair from prolonged use of personal stereo headphones. {Journal of the American Medical Association, 1984}

(Allergy to headphones. Treat with NAET; avoid 24 hours)

ANCHORMAN GLAZE:

Glazed-eye look of TV anchorman caused by looking at the teleprompter through glaring camera lights. {Syracuse, New York, TV station, 1960}

(Allergy to eye positioning. Treat with NAET. Avoid 24 hours)

ARCTIC TEMPER:

Extreme irritability developing amongst arctic explorers exposed to darkness, monotony, isolation and sensory depravation. {Lancet, 1910}

(Allergy to darkness. Treat with NAET to B vitamins, serotonin, melatonin, sunlight, loneliness.)

BEER DRINKERS FINGER:

Swelling, bluish discoloration and wasting of finger caused by placing pop-top beer can rings on finger. {JAMA, 68}

(Allergy to vitamin C, vitamin B, sugar, yeast, beer, and tin. Treat all of these with NAET)

BINGO BRAIN:

The headache associated with carbon monoxide intoxication which occurs after spending long hours in smoke filled bingo halls. {Canadian Medical Association, 1982}

(Allergy to carbonmoxide. Treat with NAET for CO)

BIRDWATCHERS TWITCH:
The nervous excitement of spotting a species for the first time.
{New Scientist, 1982}

(Allergy to B vitamins. Treat with NAET and supplement)

CHRISTMAS DEPRESSION:
Psychological stress during holidays related to the use of
alcohol and social pressures. {JAMA, 1982}
**(Allergy to turkey, serotonin, chocolate, sugar, alcohol
and the Christmas tree. Treat all of the above with
NAET.)**

CREDIT-CARD-ITIS:
Pain over the rear and down thigh due to pressure on nerve
from a wallet stuffed with credit cards. {New England Medical
Journal, 1966}
**(Allergy to leather, vinyl, plastics, credit cards, wallet.
treat all with NAET)**

DISCO DIGIT:
A sore finger from snapping fingers while dancing. {New
England Medical Journal}
**(Allergy to calcium, motion of snapping fingers. Treat with
NAET.)**

DOG WALKERS ELBOW:
Pain caused by constant tension and tugs from a dog leash.
{New England Medical Journal, 1979}

(Allergy to dog and dog leash)

ELECTRONIC SPACE-WAR VIDEO-GAME EPI-LEPSY:
Epilepsy caused by the flashing lights of electronic video games. {BMA Journal, 1982}

(Allergy to electronic radiation. Treat with NAET for B vitamins, radiation, flashing lights)

ESPRESSO WRIST:
Pain in espresso coffee machine operators from strong wrist motions required to make the coffee. {JAMA, 1956}

(Allergic to calcium, coffee, and motion)

FLIP-FLOP DERMATITIS:
Skin disease on feet from wearing rubber flip-flops. {BMA Journal, 1965}

(Allergy to the material of Flip-flop footwear. Treat with NAET for the material)

FRISBEE FINGER:
Cutting of finger from strenuous throwing of a frisbee. {New England Medical Journal, 1975}

(Allergy to frisbee. Treat with NAET to frisbee and frisbee throwing)

GOLF ARM:
Shoulder and elbow pain after too many rounds of golf. {BMA Journal, 1896}

(Allergy to golf club, ball, and motion. Treat with NAET)

HOOKERS ELBOW:
Painful shoulder swelling suffered by fishermen repeatedly jerking upwards on a fishing line. {New England Medical Journal, 1981}

(Allergy to fish, ocean air, salt, fishing net, rod and jerking motion)

HOUSWIFITIS:
Nervous symptoms related to spending too much time managing a busy household. {Centrescope, 1976}

(Allergy to household chemicals causing nervousness and brain fatigue and physical fatigue. Treat each one of the chemicals individually.)

HUMPERS LUMP:
Swelling suffered by hotel porters from lugging heavy bags. {Diseases of Occupations, 1975}

(Allergy to calcium, minerals, leather, vinyl, plastics, bags and bag lugging mtion. Treat with NAET for each item)

ICE-CREAM FROSTBITE:
Frostbite on the lips from prolonged contact with ice-cream. {New England Medical Journal, 1982}

(Allergy to vitamin C and cold. Treat with NAET)

JEANS FOLLICULITIS:
Irritation of the hair follicles from the waist down to the knees caused by ultra-tight jeans. {New England Medical Journal, 1981}

(Allergy to vitamin C, calcium and pressure. Treat each one with NAET and supplement with the vitamins)

LABEL LICKERS TONGUE:
Ulcers in mouth from sensitivity to sticky labels. {Dangerous Trades, 1902}

(Allergy to glue. Treat it with NAET)

MONEY COUNTERS CRAMP:
Painful seizure of muscles from counting too much cash. {English University Press, 1975}

(Allergy to money. Treat it with NAET)

NUNS KNEE:
Swelling of kneecap from repeated kneeling in prayer. {Diseases of Occupations, 1975}

(Allergy to calcium, vitamin C, the wood or tile or the surface where kneeling. Treat each one separately with NAET).

PANTIE GIRDLE SYNDROME:
Tingling or swelling of feet from wearing a too-tight pantie girdle. {BMA Journal, 1972}

(Allergy to elastic, pantie girdle and pressure. Treat them with NAET)

RETIRED HUSBAND SYNDROME:
Tension, headaches, depression and anxiety felt by women whose husbands have just retired. {Western Journal of Medicine, 1984}

(Allergy to the husband, B vitamins, calcium and serotonin. Treat each one and supplement the vitamins)

SEAMSTRESSES BOTTOM:
Hardening of skin following long-term trauma of rocking on the hips while operating a sewing machine. {American Family Physician, 1979}

(Allergy to vitamin C, calcium and rocking motion. treat each one and supplement the vitamins)

SICK SANTAS SYNDROME:
Back pain from lifting heavy children and parcels and acquired illnesses from multiple contact with kids. {JAMA, 1986}

(Allergy to calcium, kids, parcel -wrap materials, and lifting. Treat each one and supplement with the vitamins)

TOILET SEAT DERMATITIS:
Skin irritation on rear from spending too much time on the toilet. {Archive of Dermatology, 1933}

(Allergy to food eaten through the day and toilet seat. Treat them with NAET)

UNIFORM RASH:
Skin irritation of neck, chest and arms from wearing new uniforms. {BMJ, 1973}

(Allergy to the new material, chemical used on the material. Treat them with NAET, wash the clothes before wearing)

WORKING WIFE SYNDROME:
Fatigue, irritability, headaches and diminished sex drive from strain of doing two jobs. {Lancet, 1966}

(Allergy to adrenals, adrenaline, neurotransmitters, foods eaten regularly, fabrics worn regularly, other products used regularly, dry clean chemicals, other soaps, detergents and chemicals used in cleaning clothes, and the emotion of having to work at two jobs while others in her sitiation are working at one job)

Resources

www.naet.com - The NAET website for information regarding NAET

Nambudripad Allergy Research Foundation (NARF)
6714 Beach Blvd.
Buena Park, CA 90621
(714) 523-0800
A Nonprofit foundation dedicated to NAET research

NAET Seminars
6714 Beach Blvd.
Buena Park, CA 90621
(714) 523-8900
NAET Seminar information

Delta Publishing Company (for Books on NAET)
6714 Beach Blvd.
Buena Park, CA 90621
(714) 523-0800
E-mail: naet@earthlink.net

Jacob Teitelbaum MD
CFS/Fibromyalgia Therapies
Author of the best selling book:
"From Fatigued to Fantastic!" and

"Three Steps to Happiness! Healing Through Joy"
(410) 573-5389
www.EndFatigue.com

Environmentally Safe Products

Quantum Wellness Center

Drs. Dave & Steven Popkin

1261 South Pine Island Rd.

Plantation, FL 33324

(954) 370-1900/ Fax: (954) 476-6281

E-mail: buddha327@aol.com

Cotton Gloves and other Environmentally

Safe Health Products

Janice Corporation

198 US Highway 46

Budd Lake, NJ 07828-3001

(800) 526-4237

Herbal Supplements

Kenshin Trading Corporation
1815 West 213th Street, Ste. 180
Torrance, CA 90501
(310) 212-3199

Phenolics

Frances Taylor/Dr. Jacqueline Krohn
Los Alamos Medical Center, Ste.136
3917 West Road
Los Alamos, NM 87544
(505) 662-9620

Enzyme Formulations, Inc
6421 Enterprise Lane
Madison, WI 53719

(800) 614-4400

Allergies Lifestyle & Health
205 Center Street, Ste. B.
Eatonville, WA 98328
(360) 832-0858
Health Products

Bio Meridian
12411 S. 265 W. Ste. F
Draper, UT 84020
(801) 501-7517
Computerized Allergy Testing Services

Star Tech Health Services, LLC
1219 South 1840 West
Orem, Utah 84058
(888) 229-1114
Computerized Allergy Testing Services

Thorne Research Inc.
P.O. Box 25
Denver, ID 83825
(208) 263-1337
Herbs and Vitamins

Earth Calm
3805 Windermere Lane
Oroville, CA 95965
(530) 534 9982

Dreamous Corporation
12016 Wilshire Blvd. # 8
Los Angeles, CA 90025
(310) 442 8544

K & T Books
LAMC, Ste. 136,
3917 West Road
Los Alamos, NM 87544
(505) 662 9620

Neuropathways EEG Imaging
427 North Canon Dr. # 209
Beverly Hills, CA 90210
(310) 276 9181

CHI/KHT
P.O. Box 5309
Hemet, CA 92544
(909) 766 1426
Health Products

Biochemical Laboratories
P.O.Box 157
Edgewood, NM 87015
(800) 545 6562

Green Healing Center C
1700 Sansom St., Ste.800
Philadelphia, PA 19103
215-751-9833

BIBLIOGRAPHY

Abehsera, Michel, Ed., *Healing Ourselves,* 1973

Ali, Majid M.D., *The Canary and Chronic Fatigue,* Life Span Press, 1995

American Medical Association Committee on Rating of Mental and Physical Impairments, *Guides to the Evaluation of Permanent Impairment,* N.P., 1971

American Psychiatric Association, *Diagnostic and Statistical Manual of Mental Disorders,* 4th. ed., 2000

Andress, E. and J. Harrison. 1999. *Flavored Vinegars. In 'So Easy to Preserve'.* 4th Ed. Cooperative Extension Service, The University of Georgia. 140-143.

Austin, Mary, *Acupuncture Therapy,* 1972

Baxter, R. and W. Holzapfel. 1982. A microbial investigation of selected spices, herbs, and additives in South Africa. J. Food Sc. 47:570-574.

Beckmann, G, D. Koszegi, B. Sonnenschein and R. Leimbeck. 1996. On the microbial status of herbs and spices. Fleischwirtschaft. 76(3): 240-243.

Beeson, Paul B., M.D. and McDermott, Walsh, M.D., Eds., *Textbook of Medicine,* 12th edition, 1967

Bender, David, and Bruno Leone, *The Environment, Opposing Viewpoints,* Greenhaven Press, 1996

Blum, Jeanne Elizabeth, *Woman Heal Thyself,* Charles E. Tuttle Co., 1995

Brodal, A., M.D., *Neurological Anatomy in Relation to Clinical Medicine,* 2nd ed.

Brownstein, David, "*Overcoming Arthritis*" Medical Alternatives press, 2001

Brownstein, David, "*Hormones and Chronic Disease*" Medical Alternatives press, 1999

Brownstein, David, "*The Miracle of Natural Hormones*, 1998. 152pp. Medical Alternatives Press. Author: *The Miracle of Natural Hormones* 2nd Edition. 1999. Medical Alternatives Press

Cecil Textbook Of Medicine, 21st ed., 2000

Cerrat, Paul L., *"Does Diet Affect the Immune System?"* RN, Vol. 53, pp. 67-70 (June 1990)

Chaitow, Leon, *The Acupuncture Treatment of Pain,* Thomsons Publishers, 1984

Chernoff, Marilyn, Daily dose of toxin,1924 Juan Tabo NE, Ste A, Albuquerque, NM 87112, 2006

Collins, Douglas, R. M.D., *Illustrated Diagnosis of Systematic Diseases,* 1972

Cousins, Norman, *Head First, The Biology of Hope and the Healing Power of the Human Spirit,* Penguin Books, 1990

Daniels, Lucille, M.A, and Catherine Wothingham, Ph.D., *Muscle Testing Techniques of Manual Examination,* 3rd ed., 1972

Davis, Rowland H., and Weller, Stephen G., *The Gist of Genetics,* Jones and Bartlett Publishers, 1996

East Asian Medical Studies Society, *Fundamentals of Chinese Medicine,* Paraadigm Publications, 1985

Elliot, Frank, A., F.R.C.P., *Clinical Laboratory*, 1959

Fazir, Claude A., M.D., *Parents Guide to Allergy in Children,* Doubleday & Co., 1973

FDA - CFSAN. 1998. *Guide to minimize microbial food safety hazards for fresh fruits and vegetables. At* http://www.cfsan.fda.gov/~dms/prodguid.html.

Fratkin, Jake, *Chinese Herbal Pattent Formulas,* Institute of Traditional Medicine, 1986

Fujihara, Ken and Hays, Nancy, *Common Health Complaints,* Oriental Healing Arts Institute, 1982

Fulton, Shaton, *The Allergy Self Help Book,* Rodale Books, 1983

Gabriel, Ingrid, *Herb Identifier and Handbook,* Sterling Publishing Co., 1980

Gach, Michael Reed, *Acuppressure's Potent Points,* Bantam Books, 1990

Goldberg, Burton and Eds. of Alternative Medicine Digest, *Chronic Fatigue and Fibromyalgia & Environmental Illness*, Future Medicine Publishing, 1998

Goldberg, Burton and Eds. of Alternative Medicine Digest, *Definitive Guide to Headaches,* Future Medicine Publishing, 1997

Golos, Natalie, and Frances, *Coping With Your Allergies,* Simon and Schuster

Goodheart, George, J., *Applied Kinesiology,* N.P., 1964

---. *Applied Kinesiology*, 1970 Research Manual, 8th ed. N.P., 1971

---. *Applied Kinesiology*, 1973 Research Manual, 9th ed. N.P., 1973

---. *Applied Kinesiology*, 1974 Research Manual, N.P., 1974

---.*Applied Kinesiology*, Workshop Manual, N.P., 1972

Gray, Henry, F.R.S., *Anatomy of the Human Body,* 27th, 34th, and 38th eds., 1961

Graziano, Joseph, *Footsteps to Better Health*, N.P., 1973

Guyton, Arthur C., *Textbook of Medical Physiology,* 2nd ed., 1961

Haldeman, Scott, *Modern Developments in the Principles and Practice of Chiropractic,* Appleton-Century-Crofts, 1980

Hansel, Tim, *When I Relax I Feel Guilty,* Chariot Victor Publishing, 1979

Harris H. M.D., and Debra Fulghum Bruce, *The Fibromyalglia Handbook*, Holt and Co., 1996

Hepler, Opal, E., Ph.D., M.D., *Manual of Clinical Laboratory Methods,* 4th ed., 1962

Heuns, Him-Che., *Handbook of Chinese Herbs and Formulae,* Vol V., 1985

Bibliography

Hsu, Hong-Yen, Ph.D., *Chinese Herb Medicine and Therapy*, Oriental Healing Arts Institute, 1982

---. *Commonly Used Chinese Herb Formulas with Illustrations*, Oriental Healing Arts Institute, 1982

---. *Natural Healing With Chinese Herbs*, Oriental Healing Arts Institute, 1982

Janeway, Charles A., and Travers, Paul, and Walport, Mark, and Shlomchik, Mark, *Immunobiology*, Garland Publishing, 2001

Jusleh, R. and R. Deibel. 1974. Microbial profile of selected spices and herbs at import. J. Milk Food Technol. 37 (8): 414-419.

Kandel, Schwartz, Jessell, *Principles of Neural Science*, McGraw Hill, 4th ed., 2000

Kennington & Church, *Food Values of Portions Commonly Used*, J.B. Lippincott Company, 1998

Kirschmann J.D. with Dunne, L.J., *Nutrition Almanac*, 2nd ed., McGraw Hill Book Co., 1984

Krohn, Jacqueline, M.D., and Taylor, Frances A., M.A. and Larson, Erla Mae, R.N., *Allergy Relief and Prevention*, 2nd ed., Hartley & Marks, 1996

Krohn, Jacqueline, M.D., and Taylor, Frances A., M.A., *Natural Detoxification*, 2nd ed., Hartley & Marks, 2000

Lawson-Wood, Denis, F.A.C.A. and Lawson-Wood, Joyce, *The Five Elements of Acupuncture and Chinese Massage*, 2nd ed., 1973

Lyght, Charles E., M.D., and John M. Trapnell, M.D., Eds., *The Merck Manual,* 11th ed., Merck Research Laboratories, 1966

MacKarness, Richard, *The Hazards of Hidden Allergies,* Mc Ilwain

Merkel, Edward K., and John, David T., and Krotoski, Wojciech A., Eds., Medical Parasitology, 8th. ed., W.B.Saunders Company, 1999

Milne, Robert, M.D., and More, Blake, and Goldberg, Burton, An Alternative Medicine Definitive Guide to Headaches, 1997

Mindell, Earl, Vitamin Bible, Warner Books, 1985.

Moss, Louis, M.D., Acupuncture and You, 1964

Moyers, Bill, Healing and the Mind, Doubleday, 1976

Nambudripad, DS: *NAET® Protocols and Procedures-part 1,* The Journal of NAET Energetics and Complementary Medicine, 2005, Vol. (1) (1), pp.17-25.NAET Center, Buena Park, CA, 2005.

Nambudripad, DS: *NAET® Protocols and Procedures-part 2,* The Journal of NAET Energetics and Complementary Medicine, 2005, Vol. (1)(2), pp.107-112.NAET Center, Buena Park, CA.

Nambudripad, DS: *NAET® Protocols and Procedures-part 3,* The Journal of NAET Energetics and Complementary Medicine, Vol. (1)(3), pp.179-184. NAET Center, Buena Park, CA, 2005.

Nambudripad, DS: *NAET® Protocols and Procedures-part 4,* The Journal of NAET Energetics and Complementary Medi-

Bibliography

cine, 2005, Vol. (1) (4), pp.265-270. NAET Center, Buena Park, CA.

Nambudripad, DS: *NAET® Protocols and Procedures-part 5*, The Journal of NAET Energetics and Complementary Medicine, Vol. (2)(1), pp.343-350. NAET Center, Buena Park, CA, 2005.

Nambudripad, Devi, *Living Pain Free*, Delta Publishing Company, 1997

Nambudripad, Devi, *Say Good-bye to ADD and ADHD*, Delta Publishing Company, 1999

Nambudripad, Devi, *Say Good-bye to Allergy-related Autism*, Delta Publishing Company, 1999

Nambudripad, Devi, *Say Good-bye to Children's Allergies*, Delta Publishing Company, 2000

Nambudripad, Devi, *Say Good-bye to Environmental Allergies*, Delta Publishing Company, 2002

Nambudripad, Devi, *Say Good-bye to Chemical Sensitivities*, Delta Publishing Company, 2002

Nambudripad, Devi, *Surviving Biohazard Agents*, Delta Publishing Company, 2002

Nambudripad, Devi, *The NAET Guidebook*, Delta Publishing Company, 2001

Northrup, Christiane M.D., *Women's Bodies, Women's Wisdom*, Bantam Books, 1998

Palos, Stephan, *The Chinese Art of Healing*, 1972

Pearson, Durk, and Shaw, Sandy, *The Life Extension Companion,* Warner Books, 1984

Pert, Candace B., Ph.D., *Molecules of Emotion,* Scribner, 1997

Pitchford, Paul, *Healing with Whole Foods,* North Atlantic Books, 1993

Powers, E., R. Lawyer and Y. Masuoka. 1975. *Microbiology of Processed spices. J. Milk Food Technol.* 39 (11): 683-687.

Radetsky, Peter, *Allergic to the Twentieth Century,* Boston, Little, Brown and Co., 1997

Randolph, Theron, G., M.D., and Ralph W. Moss, Ph.D., *An Alternative Approach to Allergies,* Lippincott and Conwell, 1980

Rapp, Doris, *Allergy and Your Family,* Sterling Publishing Co., 1980

Rapp, Doris, *Is This Your Child?* Quill, William Morrow, 1991

Shanghai College of Traditional Chinese, *Acupuncture, a Comprehensive Text*

Shealy, C. Norman, M.D., Ph. D. and Caroline Myss, Ph. D., *The Creation of Health,* Stillpoint Publishing, 1993

Shima, Mike, *The Medical I Ching,* Blue Poppy Press, 1992

Shubert, Charlotte "Burned by FlameRretardants?" SCIENCE NEWS Vol. 160 (October 13, 2001), pgs. 238-239.

Sierra, Ralph, U., *Chiropractic Handbook of Applied Neurology,* Mexico, 1956

Somekh, Emile, M.D. *The Complete Guide To Children's Allergies,*   Pinnacle Books, Inc. 1979

Smith, CW, Electromagnetic Man: *Health and Hazard in the Electrical Environment*, Martin's Press, 1989, 90, 97

Smith CW,   Environmental Medicine: *Electromagnetic Aspects of Biological Cycles,* 1995:9(3):113-118

Smith CW., *Electrical Environmental Influences on the Autonomic Nervous System,* 11th. Intl. Symp. on *"Man and His Environment in Health and Disease"*, Dallas, Texas, February 25-28,1993

Smith CW., *Electromagnetic Fields and the Endocrine System,* 10th. Intl. Symp. on *"Man and His Environment in Health and Disease"*, Dallas Texas, February 27- March 1, 1992

Smith CW., *Basic Bioelectricity: Bioelectricity and Environmental Medicine,* 15th. Intl. Symp., on *"Man and His Environment in Health and Disease",* Dallas, Texas, February 20-23, 1997. (Audio Tapes from: Professional Audio Recording, 2300 Foothill Blvd. #409, La Verne, CA

Smith, John, H., D.C., *Applied Kinesiology and the Specific Muscle Balancing Technique.*

J.E. Teitelbaum, B. Bird, R.M. Greenfield, et al., *"Effective Treatment of CFS and FMS: A Randomized, Double-Blind Placebo Controlled Study,"* Journal of Chronic Fatigue Syndrome 8 (2) (2001).

Teitlebaum, Jacob, M.D.,*Three Steps to Happiness!* 1st ed., 2001, Avery Penguin Putnam

Teitlebaum, Jacob, M.D.,*Healing through Joy"* 1st ed., 2002, Avery Penguin Putnam

Teitlebaum, Jacob, M.D.,*Pain Pain Go Away* !1st ed., 2003, 2nd. ed., 2001, Avery Penguin Putnam

Sui, Choa Kok, *Pranic Healing*, Samuel Wiser, 1990

Weiss, Jordan, M.D., *Psychoenergetics,* 2nd. ed., Oceanview Publishing, 1995

Zong, Linda, *"Chinese Internal Medicine,"* lectures at SAMRA University, Los Angeles, 1985

Case Histories from the Author's private practice,1984-present

Index

A

A Collection of NAET® Cases 207
A tip to master self-testing 153
Abdominal bloating 165
About person-to-person allergies 156
Acetic acid 95
Acupuncture 19
Acute care 203
Acutherapy 198
Adrenal depletion 57
Agar 95
Alcat test 105
Alcohol 181
Aldicarb 95, 96
Alginates 95, 96
Allergic rhinitis 62
Allergic to cotton 218
Allergic to other human beings 57
Allergies to people 188
Allergy elimination 19
Allergy relief, finally 224
Allergy sympom checklist 33
Allergy to perfume 220
Allergy to slim fast 222

Aluminum salts 95, 96, 97
Amino acids 2 182
Amino acids-1 182
Amygdala 11
Anaphylactic shock 72, 79
Anesthesia 82
Animal fats 182
Ant spray on the newspaper 223
Antibodies 27
Antigens 14
Arthritis 73
Artificial sweeteners 181
Artificial sweeteners 72
Asking questions 158
Asthma 64
Asthma 71
Asthma 90
Athlete's foot 85
Attraction 25
Autistic behaviors 74

B

B complex 177
Backache 205
Bad breath 165
Baking powder 184
Banana 72
Basal ganglia 11

Base 179
BBF treatment 176
Bell pepper and asthma 236
Benzoates 95
Beverages 70
Biochemistry 18
Blood pressure test 106
Bradykinin 13
Breast abscesses 73
Bronchial asthma 84, 239
Bronchial asthma and body ache 235

C

Cal. Proprionate 95, 97
Cal. Silicate 95, 98
Calcium 176
Camillo golgi 10
Cancer 90
Carbamates 95, 98
Carbon monoxide 98
Carbon monoxide poisoning 215
Career-produced allergies 78
Casein 98
Categories of allergens 59
Categories of allergies 56
Causes of chemical sensitivities 4
Central nervous system 11
Cerebral cortex 9
Cervical cancer 78
Cesarean section 82
Chalk powder 63
Chemical mediator 27
Chemical sprays, 63
Chemicals 179

Chemicals from printing shop 221
Chiropractic 19
Chiropractor xv
Choking 68
Chronic sinusitis 164
Cigarette smell 69
Cigarette smoking 69
Classic naet group 193
Claude bernard 11
Chlorox 179
Coffee mix 181
Combination allergies 58
Commonly seen emotional blockages 205
Condiments 70
Contactants 59, 76
Cooking pans induced disorders 67
Cooks 78
Corn mix 182
Cotton 56
Cough variant asthma 66
Crude oil 193
Crude oils 78

D

Depressed immune system 5
Depression 76
Dermatitis 64
Detecting allergies 89
Detergents 191
Diabetes 57
Diphtheria 84
Dominating energy 146
Dr. Albert H. Rowe 106

Heredity 4
Hereditary 6
Heavy metals 181
Hearing loss 57
He was anaphylactic peanuts 236
Hay-fever 62
Hair and nails 57

H

Gymnasium 85
Gutta percha tissue 91
Gum mix 185
Grapefruit 73
Grain mix 178
Glutamate 13
Genetic factors 59
Genetic causes 83
Gelatin 185
Galen 10

G

Frequent colds 165
Formic acid 95, 99
Foods 70
Food colors 180
Food chemicals 94
Food bleach 95, 99
Food additives 180
Fluoride 186
Flowers 57
Fish mix 185
Fibrocystic breasts 78
Fever 205
Feminine tampons 78

Feces 57
Feathers 92, 93
Fear triggered his asthma 238
Fatigue 164, 205
Family history 91
Fainting 205

F

Fabrics 183

Exposure xiii
Exercise xiii
Excessive thirst, 132
Excessive hunger 132
Epstein-barr virus 84
Environmentally ill 218
Enterovirus 98
Energy flow through 12 meridians 108
Energy boosting techniques 188
Emphysema, 69, 70
Emotions 18
Emotional traumas 5
Emotional stressors 59, 86
Emotional allergies 58
Emotional allergies 188
Electro magnetic field test 103
Electrical signals 11
Egg mix 176
EDTA 95, 98
Eczema 74, 163

E

Dynamometer testing 102
Drugs given in infancy 183
Dried bean mix 182

Hermann von helmholtz 10
Hippocampus 11
Histamine 13
History 101
Hives 74
Hold, sit and test 194
Hold, sit and wait 104
Home evaluation procedures 28
Hormones 179
Hot flashes 83
House dust 63
How was naet® discovered 20
Hyperactivity 74, 165
Hypo-functioning immune systems 83
Hypothalamus 14, 18

I

I am enjoying my life again! 229
I handled my weight problem through naet® 228
I was allergic to my nasal spray 238
I was anaphylactic to shellfish 233
Ice cream 83
Immune system mediators 13
Immunizations 81
Immunoglobulins 26
Indoor plants 93
Infectants 59, 80
Infections 4
Influenza 91
Ingestants 59, 70
Inhalants 59, 188
Inheritance 27
Injectants 59, 79
Insect bites 187
Intradermal test 106
Irish whiskey 73
Iron mix 177
Irritability 74
Irritation and fatigue from eating products 87
Isolating the blockages 197
Italian physician 10

J

Johannes Muller 10
John Langley 11
Joint pains and arthritis 164

K

Kidney failure 57
Kinesiology 19
Kittens - case study 215

L

Large intestine channel (meridian) 113
Latex products 187
Leather xliii, xlv
Lethal bites 80
Leukotrienes 13
Liver failure 57
Luigi Galvani 10
Lung channel 111

Lung meridian-essential nutrition 110, 114, 117, 120, 122, 126, 128

Lupus 76

Lupus erythematosus 73

M

M.C.S - case study 208

Magnesium silicate 100

Malabsorption 5

Malic acid 99

Mannan 99

Mannitol 99

Mast cells 13

Medulla 9

Meridians 86

Migraine 164

Milk 176

Milk-albumin 95

Mineral mix 178

Miracle in the mountains 212

Molds and fungi 84

Molds and fungi 599

NST 102

MSG 93, 181

MSG Sensitivity 1

Multiple Chemical Sensitivities 210

Multiple chemical sensitivity 58

Multiple sclerosis 73, 82

My Chronic Cough 234

My Nasal spray 236

N

NAET® xxiii, 8, 19, 64, 101

NAET® Basic Allergens 174

NAET® intervention 15

NAET® made lives worth living 227

NAET® rotation diet 104

NAET ®Self-Testing procedure 193

NAET® testing procedures 141

NAET®-QRT Procedure 157

NAET® has given me my life back! 239

NAETER 102

Names of the Meridians 30

Nasal mucosa 14

Nasal polyps, 63

Naugahyde 78

Nausea 205

Nerve cells 14

Neuro Muscular Sensitivity Testing 143

Neuropeptides 12

Neurotransmitters 181

Newspaper ink, 63

Night shade vegetables 186

No More Anaphylactic Reactions 232

No more nasal Infection 237

Normal Energy Flow 108

NST procedure 143

NST with allergen 148

NST without allergen 144

NST-NAET ® 143

Nut Mix 1 84

Nut Mix 2 184

Nutrition 19

O

Orange 72

Organ failure 57

Organ-Meridian Association Time 29
Organic chemical water pollutants: 101
Organization 9
Other chemical agents 189
Other Hormones 184
Oval Ring Test 149
Overview of NAET® 21

P

Paper products 185
Parasympathetic 12
Paul ehrlich in germany 11
Peanuts 72
Perfume 184,, 208
Peripheral endings 12
Personal clothing 192
Pesticides 186
Pesticides 75
Physical agents 82
Physical agents 59
Physical examination 102
Plastics 183
Pollens 64
Pons 9
Poor vision 57
Posttraumatic disorders 5
Professional singer 87
Propylene glycol 96
Prostaglandins 13
Pulse test 1033

Q

Question response Testing 156

R

Radiation 5, 187
Ramon Y Cajal 10
RAST 106
Raynaud's disease 83
Refined starches 183
Repulsion 25
Respiratory distress 80
Resuscitation points 203
Rheumatic fever 84
Rheumatism 90
Root canal 91

S

Sage weeds 62
Salicylic acid 99
Saliva 57
Salt mix 178
Santiago 10
Scaly skin 164
School work materials 183
Sciatica 73
Scratch test 106
Sea of energy 146
Seasonal allergic rhinitis 62
Secretin 95, 100
Semen 57
Sense organs 11
Shellfish mix 185
Silk 56
Skin lesions 83
Smoke 193
Sodium aluminum phosphate 96
Spice mix 184
Spleen channel 118, 119
Sports-related injury 71

Index

Stomach acid 179
Stomach meridian 115
Storing the memory 11
Substance p 13
Succinic acid 95
Sugar mix 177
Surrogate testing 154
Sweat 57
Sympathetic nerves 12
Symptoms of meridians 107
Synapse 14
Synthetic bra 78

T

Talc 100
Tartaric acid 100
Tears 57
Temporal lobe 18
Tendency 6
Tequila 73
Testing person-to-person allergies 156
Testing through an extended surrogate 154
Tetanus antitoxin 90
Thalamus 9, 18
The pericardium meridian 129
The association cortex 12
The basis of NAET® 18
The brain 9
The brain and allergies 11
The brain and the nervous system 8
The cerebellum 9
The communication network 13
The conception vessel meridian 138, 139

The end of my sensitivities 219
The gall bladder meridian 133, 134
The governing vessel meridian 137, 139
The heart meridian 121, 122
The kidney meridian 127, 128
The large intestine meridian 112, 113
The liver meridian 135, 136
The lung meridian 109, 111
The midbrain 9
The nervous system 8, 10
The oriental medicine CPR point 203
The pericardium meridian 129, 130
The sensory cortex 11
The small intestine meridian 123, 124
The spleen meridian 118, 119
The stomach meridian 116
The techniques of asking questions 159
The triple warmer meridian 131, 132
The ultimate technique 214
Thyroid 57
Tissues and secretions 188
Toxins 4
Treating by priority 192
Trigeminal neuralgia 73
Tryptophane 13
Tuberculosis 84, 90
Turkey 181
Twenty-first century xxiii, 7

U

Universal reactors 58
Urinary bladder meridian
125, 126

V

Vaccinations 5, 81, 183
Vegetable fats 182
Vertigo 73
Vital signs 102
Vitamin A 177
Vitamin C 177
Vitamin C induced body ache!
226
Vitamin D 186
Vitamin E 186
Vitamin F 182
Vitamin K 186

W

Wasp 79
Water chemicals 100, 207
Water filtering system "Culligan"
207
Water pollutants 100, 207
What is chemical sensitivity 47
What is multiple chemical
sensitivity 48
What is NAET® 19
What is sinusitis? 65
Whey 185
Whiten all 180
Woolen clothes 77
Wrought-iron 76

Y

Yeast infections 85
Yeast mix 178
Yeast-like infection 165
Yogurt 1855

BOOK ORDER FORM

Name of book	Price	Quantity	Total Price
Say Good-bye to Illness			
3rd. Edition (English)	$24.00	------------	--------------
Spanish Edition	$21.00	------------	--------------
French Edition	$24.00	------------	--------------
German Edition	$24.00	------------	--------------
Japanese Edition	$24.00	------------	--------------
Say Good-bye to ADD & ADHD	$18.00	------------	--------------
Freedom From Environmental Sensitivities	$18.00	------------	--------------
Freedom From Chemical Sensitivities	$18.00	------------	--------------
Say Good-bye to allery-related Autism-2nd ed.	$18.00	------------	--------------
Say Good-bye to Children's Allergies	$18.00	------------	--------------
Say Good-bye to Your Allergies	$18.00	------------	--------------
Say Good-bye to Asthma	$18.00	------------	--------------
Say Good-bye to Headaches	$18.00	------------	--------------
Say Goodbye to Bipolar Disease	$18.00	------------	--------------
NAET Guide Book, 6th Ed.	$12.00	------------	--------------
Living Pain Free	$22.95	------------	--------------

Sales Tax	---------
S&H	---------
Total	---------

To order books, call:

(714) 523-8900 or (888) 890-0670

or send a check for the amount plus the applicable sales tax
and $5.00 for shipping and handling to:

Delta Publishing Company
6714 Beach Blvd.
Buena Park, CA 90621

Or vist the website: www.naet.com